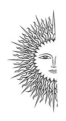

YONDERCOTT
PRESS

A Guide to
Homeopathic
First Aid

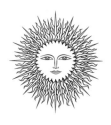

YONDERCOTT
PRESS

Written by the School of Homeopathy · wwwhomeopathyschool.com
Illustrated by Jenny Grist, Terry Harris & Amanda Norland
© 1990 - 2015 The School of Homeopathy. All rights reserved

1st Edition edited by Mary Castle and Vanessa Hope, published 1990
2nd Edition published 1991
3rd Edition revised by Misha Norland & Julia Hunn, published 1996
4th Edition revised by Misha Norland & Mani Norland, published 2006
5th Edition revised by Misha Norland & Mani Norland, published 2010
6th Edition revised by Misha Norland & Mani Norland, published 2015

Published by Yondercott Press
Orchard Leigh, Rodborough Hill, Stroud, Gloucestershire, GL5 3SS, UK
© Yondercott Press 2015
ISBN 978-0-9544766-3-2
www.yondercottpress.com

British Library Cataloguing in Publishing Data
A catalogue record for this book is available from the British Library.

This book contains general information only. The authors accept no liability for injury,
loss or damage to anyone acting on the contents of this book. No responsibility is
accepted for any errors or omissions in the contents of the book.

Contents

Introduction

Prescribing and dispensing

Index to common ailments

Remedies

Further information

Introduction

Welcome To Homeopathic First Aid Prescribing

Since you are reading this, it follows that you want to treat accidents and common ailments as quickly, effectively and safely as possible. We are sure that health and happiness are high on your list of priorities for all your family. Homeopathy can offer effective self-help because it stimulates your body's innate capacity for self-healing. When you take homeopathic medicines (remedies) you should experience, not only quick and effective relief of acute suffering, but also an increase in wellbeing. Over time and with continued treatment you should also notice a decreasing tendency to fall ill.

This book is a basic and practical introduction to homeopathy. We recommend that you seek to inform yourself further, and perhaps consult an experienced homeopath if you intend to make long-term changes in your health habits or move away from a reliance on conventional medication. Whilst homeopathy can promote healing on a great many levels, we respect medical science and know that there is a case for conventional treatment for conditions with developed pathology and, of course, surgical intervention may be necessary for emergency situations. The two systems of medicine each have their part to play, and the authors of this booklet look forward to the time when each not only endorse the other, but fully cooperate to deliver the finest health-care.

What Is Homeopathy?

Homeopathy is a holistic method of overcoming sickness and promoting long-term wellbeing. It takes into account not just the physical, but mental and emotional symptoms too as they are all expressions of the body's distress. It is only when you lose your ability to rebalance yourself that your being responds by evolving symptoms. These are the outward signs of an internal disturbance. Homeopaths seek to understand diseases by viewing all of your symptoms and finding their match in the form of a remedy. The remedy works by stimulating your internal energetic (spiritual) life-preserving powers (outwardly functioning through your immune defence systems) so that you return to optimum health. Many people, describing their recovery, have said that it is as though concentric rings of healing were moving outwards, from the centre to the periphery.

Individual Susceptibility

Homeopaths recognise that each individual has a different take to a similar set of circumstances. For instance, a news item depicting a plane crash may trigger heart palpitations with indignation at the perceived incompetence of the pilot in one person, or profound sadness and weeping at the fate of the passengers in a second. This also holds true even if the trigger is a common virus. For instance, a cold travelling around the neighbourhood may result in a cough and wheeziness in Mum, who is still up and about; a profuse discharge of clear running mucus in Dad, who is sneezy, weak and bedridden; the next door neighbour has thick, yellowish green mucus and is very tearful; whereas little Sally has not been touched at all, and remains happy and well. Healing is available to all who are adversely affected, and is tailored to suit each individual person, taking into account how they are experiencing their imbalance and manifesting their disease. First aid treatment looks at how a person experiences their immediate suffering, while not focusing upon the background to that suffering. Even though this 'immediate prescribing' theoretically has a limited, although positive, effect, such prescriptions can and often do touch upon the underlying state. It is astonishing how a first aid prescription can frequently improve the overall and long-term health of a person. In the later part of this booklet 'remedy pictures' are given that make reference to not only first aid symptoms, but also underlying states, to help you become familiar with a bigger picture that takes an individual's susceptibility into account.

How Does It Work?

A group of symptoms provides the essential guide to what your body needs help with. That is why homeopaths never treat isolated symptoms, or attempt to eradicate them singly. For example, a car mechanic would not knock out a flashing dashboard warning light, but would seek to understand the meaning of this and other symptoms in order to identify and then mend the broken part. Likewise, a homeopathic response is holistic: taking the parts into account to understand the whole.

The healing stimulus provided by the well selected remedy manifests in the person as a preliminary intensification (aggravation) of presenting symptoms prior to initiating healing responses. In acute and first aid situations the intensification of presenting symptoms is short lived and will usually go unnoticed. In chronic diseases, emotions, fluids, pus, and other formerly held-in states or discharges are released from within to without via the shortest venting route. The homeopath Constantine Hering (1800 – 1880) observed the following: that chronic diseases are cured in reverse chronology, the latest symptoms to have manifested are cured first, whilst the oldest symptoms are cured last of all. Disease moves out of organs of greater importance (for survival) to organs of lesser importance. During cure 'old' symptoms tend to 'move' from above to below, from central to external parts.

When you are treated homeopathically in a first aid context, the aggravation before cure will be so brief as to go unnoticed. One of the first things you should experience is that you rapidly begin feel better in yourself. Then your symptoms will recede. If you continue to have homeopathic treatment your immune responses will become stronger, and you will become less susceptible to ill health. This applies also to your emotional wellbeing, which plays an essential part in your body's susceptibility to illness in the first place. One additional, but important, point about children: they are the products of their family, which is a living organism in itself. So healthy, happy children are the outcome of healthy, happy families. For best results, we can all pull together, and this is promoted by treating all members of the family homeopathically whenever one member is out of balance.

Guidelines On What You Can Treat

You can easily treat first aid conditions such as injuries resulting from stepping on nails, cuts, minor burns etc. Also easily treatable are acute conditions with a clear causation, such as a headache after too much coffee, diarrhoea after eating rotten food. You can most successfully treat definite, unambiguous symptoms that group together and clearly indicate a remedy.

You would be well advised to get professional help when treating recurrent, chronic conditions, i.e. sets of symptoms that come back regularly, such as period pains, IBS, (Irritable Bowel Syndrome) and migraine headaches, unless you 'strike lucky' first time with your prescription. Be wary of treating people taking much medication. Steer clear of treating people with loosely defined symptoms, or where, for example, lots of things are going on at the same time, whether emotionally, mentally or physically, (unless, of course, these symptoms nonetheless cohere into a recognisable remedy picture).

You are not legally permitted to treat 'notifiable' diseases, such as, infectious childhood diseases like mumps, chickenpox, pandemics and sometimes diarrhoea (depending upon the causation). However, because you are the primary carer within your own family, you may take your child to a medical doctor immediately after you have prescribed. This gives a chance for the remedy to work before any medical interventions are needed.

The Discovery Of Homeopathy

The name homeopathy is taken from the Greek homoeos, meaning similar, and pathos, meaning suffering. It means treating the symptoms of a sick person with a substance that produces similar symptoms to those that the person is suffering from. The medicinal qualities of substances (remedies) are found by experimentation, where a trial group of healthy volunteers undergo rigorous testing. While many trace the origins of this idea to the Greek doctor and philosopher, Hippocrates (who lived 2400 years ago), it is likely that the method of cure he described originated in the African continent, since most ideas of the classical Greeks came from the temples and libraries of Egypt, especially those in Alexandria. Though it is hard to discover who first cured by homeopathic methods, there is no doubt that the sixteenth century

Swiss healer and philosopher Paracelsus and the eighteenth century German doctor Samuel Hahnemann struggled to persuade sceptics that a substance which produces symptoms in a healthy person cures those symptoms in a sick one.

Like Cures Like

When the symptom picture of the healing agent, found by experimentation, matches your diseased symptom picture, it enormously stimulates your capacity for re-balancing, helping you to do the work of 'venting' the disease symptoms and returning to health. This principle is understood in the field of everyday psychology. We know that grief (inner disturbance) is eased by tears (outward expression, symptoms), that sadness when vented does not play out as chronic brooding over the past or develop into say, anorexia, insidious weakness or MS; that anger when it is expressed does not fester and turn to hatred or develop into, say heart disease or cancer.

Samuel Hahnemann (1755 – 1843) is regarded as the father of homeopathy, and did pioneering work to provide the structured base from which we now practise, and to demonstrate that treating like with like was valid and workable. He recorded all his work in a scientific manner so that we still refer to his original experiments where he discovered the healing qualities of substances by accurately observing and recording the type of symptoms produced when a substance was given to healthy volunteers.

In the paragraph, 'What is Homeopathy?' we stated: the remedy works by stimulating your internal energetic (spiritual) life-preserving powers (outwardly functioning through your immune defence systems) so that, starting from the inside and working outward, you return to optimum health. This is how the minute, potentised and thus energetic doses act: it is because they match and resonate with your disturbed, energetic, life-preserving powers, enhancing them and your capacity for self-healing. The genius of this system of medicine is in recognising that body, feelings and mind all display what is needed; all we have to do is find a substance that mimics these symptoms and give it in small, stimulating doses Thus the body will do the rest and heals us.

Prescribing & dispensing

How Do I Prescribe?

Because homeopathy treats the person as an individual, you give a remedy according to the overall picture rather than on isolated physical symptoms alone. A brief description or picture of most of the remedies we refer to is found at the back of this booklet.

Particular attention should be paid to:
- The person's emotional state, for instance, are they irritable, anxious, weepy or lonely?
- Causative factors, for instance, have they recently had a shock, been exposed to cold and damp, fallen from a tree, or fallen out with a beloved friend?
- At which time of the day or night do they feel better or worse?
- Are they sensitive to movement, touch, pressure, noise, heat or cold?
- Are they perspiring? Which part is affected?
- Do they want hot or cold drinks, or none at all?
- What sort of food are they asking for? Have they developed an aversion to that which was previously liked?
- How did the condition develop – quickly or slowly?
- On which side of the body did the symptoms first appear,? On the right or left? Where are they now?
- What does the pain feel like? For instance, is it stinging, burning, cutting or aching?
- Do any of the symptoms appear in groups, for instance, nausea when smelling cooking, cystitis during menstruation or headache improved after urination?

Then choose the remedy picture that most closely matches the picture of the illness. Do not mix remedies. Choose the one remedy you think best matches the symptoms and only repeat the doses until improvement has been properly established, then stop. Obviously, if the remedy has no effect, even after a few repeated doses, stop giving it. Your aim is to stimulate the body. Once given the curative stimulus the body will continue the healing process by itself. Only start treatment again if the person gets worse, and then continue to give doses until improvement is once again established. See the section on, 'Dosage and Repetition'.

How To Store The Remedies

They should be stored in their original containers in a cool dry place, away from direct sunlight. They also need to be kept away from strong smells such as those given off by peppermint oil, eucalyptus oil, Tiger Balm, Vicks, and Olbas Oil.

How To Take Remedies

They need to be taken in a clean mouth, free from smoke, food or drink. It is best to avoid cleaning your teeth for at least ten minutes either before or after taking your remedy. If possible, place the remedy under the tongue, to be sucked, not swallowed. Close the lid carefully and tightly after use and put back into store.

Alternatively, the remedy can be dropped into a glass containing a couple of tablespoons of fresh water. The glass should be twirled around for a minute prior to giving the dose. It is not required that the remedy totally dissolves, as its medicinal activity will be conveyed to the water almost immediately. The water should be sipped slowly. This is of particular value when treating animals, when the water can be lapped up, or put into a clean sprayer and misted onto the animal's nose.

Dosage and Repetition

Once you have selected the remedy we suggest one pill of 30c potency should be taken and repeated every 5 to 15 minutes until definite improvement is maintained. Then you can stop taking the doses. How long it will take for improvement to be established depends on the pace of the illness. For instance, a child throwing a fever is able to respond very quickly, and thus you would expect a speedy reaction to the remedy. If the fever starts to improve quickly, but then the improvement slows down, check that the symptoms still require the original remedy and if they do, then repeat it every fifteen minutes for the next hour, or longer if necessary. If the symptoms, although less severe, continue despite the repetition of the dose, then the 200c potency of the same remedy may be used. If there is no further improvement, then another remedy should be tried, looking carefully again at the whole symptom picture.

If there is a deep wound or broken bone the healing process may take weeks so the dose should be repeated twice or thrice daily until the repair is complete. Once your health (or your patient's health) improves then stop the doses. Never try and finish a 'course' of pills. Remember homeopathic remedies are not like antibiotics where the course should be completed or relapse may occur.

ONCE YOU ARE BETTER, STOP TAKING THE REMEDIES.
IF IN DOUBT, OR IF THE SYMPTOMS DO NOT IMPROVE, PLEASE
CONTACT AN EXPERIENCED HOMEOPATH FOR HELP AND GUIDANCE.

Common Sense Measures
We wish to treat with medicines as seldom as possible, only when the body cannot cope without help. There are many other aids apart from pills that can give relief. If symptoms are mild, then these 'common sense' measures should be tried first.

ACUTE FEVER is an efficient healing process, which, as long as it is not painful, prolonged or the temperature too high, can be allowed to run its course. The function of fever is to inhibit bacterial and viral reproduction. It is an effective survival mechanism developed by mammals against infection. Medical intervention to reduce febrile response is an obvious nonsense. However, when a high temperature interferes with brain function, leading to hallucinations or convulsions, then immediate action should be taken. This is when homeopathic remedies work miracles. However, should you fail to find the right remedy, you may sponge down your patient using a bowl of cool to tepid water, concentrating on the wrists and around the neck and base of the head, to gently bring down the temperature. If fever persists, then seek professional help.

LOCAL INFLAMMATION. Sponging down an inflamed area with cool water relieves local inflammation, as does a lettuce or cabbage leaf compress, or a compress of any living greens. In the case of an abscess or boil, a compress helps to 'draw it out' and heal it. Most of us are familiar with the use of a dock leaf to relieve the pain and inflammation of being stung by nettles. This action is similar to that of any compress comprising fresh leaves. A compress may be made by loosely binding leaves to the affected area or placing a few fresh leaves within damp tea-towels on the affected part. The compress will need replacing once the leaves have lost their green colour.

HEADACHES: In these days of increasing stress headaches are common and can often be relieved by neck stretches or rolls, pressure on points at the base of the skull or neck, shoulder and head massage. If you are prone to headaches then consult a qualified homeopath for constitutional treatment.

SORE THROATS: Gargles with a mixture of salt and water, or sage tea and cider, or vinegar and honey are often sufficient to ease the pain. A dozen drops of Calendula Tincture (see Creams, Tinctures and Ointments) mixed in with the gargle will give added benefit.

NAUSEA AND VOMITING: If the condition continues for any length of time, find a homeopathic remedy, and then seek professional help. If you are worried about dehydration (losing too much fluid from the body) use a dehydration mixture of quarter of a teaspoon of salt and half a teaspoon of honey or sugar in a pint of water, a tablespoon to be taken every 15 minutes. Or for children, you can freeze fruit juice and then crush the cubes and offer one teaspoon at a time. After a bout of vomiting or diarrhoea do not eat solid food for at least 6 hours. Clear soups may be offered. Avoid milk or dairy products as the enzyme that digests milk is often destroyed during the illness and may take some time to re-establish itself. The best first food to offer is a non-fatty, easily digestible diet, such as well cooked (mushy) whole rice, steamed vegetables, porridge, bananas, and cooked apples and/or pears.

Creams, Tinctures and Ointments
PRODUCING YOUR OWN TINCTURE: Quite a few of the accident remedies grow easily in gardens, allotments and by the wayside. They are not poisons. First of all you must cross check that you indeed have the one you think you have. Google images is good for this. Then you collect all that grows above ground at the time of flowering. Cram this into a cleaned out jam-jar and top up almost to the brim with vodka. Close the lid firmly and store on a shelf where you may easily reach to give a shake daily. After six to eight weeks the liquid will be ready to pour off. This should be bottled up and stored in a cool and dark place ready for use. The tincture will need to be diluted before use. Use slightly warmed water (body heat) adding one part tincture in ten parts water.

PRODUCING DRIED HERBS AND MAKING YOUR OWN INFUSION: You may gather leaves and/or flowers, which should be collected when they are fully open in fine weather in the morning, and when the dew has been dried by the sun. Dry them quickly in the shade in a current of warm air, spreading them out on sheets of paper, without their touching each other. When they are dried, keep them in clean glass jars, stoppered against dust. When required you make an infusion of the strength of one ounce of dried leaves or flowers to a pint of freshly boiling water (you turn off the heat immediately after bringing back to the boil). This may be used when cooled. The infusion stores in a jar in the fridge for 2-3 days when a small portion may be re-heated to body temperature for use as and when.

CALENDULA OINTMENT or CREAM acts like an antiseptic and promotes healing. The ointment is excellent for cuts, grazes, chapped lips, nappy rash, cracked nipples during breast-feeding, cracked skin etc. (See the section on Cuts.)

CALENDULA TINCTURE also acts like a mild antiseptic, and diluted 1:20 in warmed water, can be used for bathing cuts and grazes. Add half a teaspoon to a cup of cooled boiled water for a mouthwash, for a sore throat or an ulcer. Use two drops in an eye bath of cooled boiled and slightly salty water (to taste like tears) if an eye is scratched. See EUPHRASIA TINCTURE below.

HYPERICUM TINCTURE and CREAM may be used in the same way when nerves are injured. It is also excellent when combined with CALENDULA for burns. Pharmacists combine the two above substances, as the injuries often accompany one another.

CANTHARIS or BURN OINTMENT if applied immediately will make the area feel hotter momentarily, but the pain and inflammation will be greatly eased within a few minutes. This initial intensification of pain is the response by the body to the action of the similar remedy. The ointment should be regularly re-applied during the next few hours. If the burns are extensive, seek medical aid, but this should not prevent you from using your remedies.

TAMUS OINTMENT is good for chilblains.

PYRETHRUM TINCTURE or SPRAY helps bites and stings.

LEDUM TINCTURE for puncture wounds from rusty nails etc., also take the remedy in pill form in 30c potency. (See the section on Wounds.)

EUPHRASIA TINCTURE for sticky, inflamed eyes. Put one or two drops in an eye-bath filled with boiled cooled water which is slightly salty (to taste like tears, see section on Eyes). If the eye is scratched, add one or two drops of CALENDULA TINCTURE. Because these are tinctures and therefore contain alcohol, it is important to use them sparingly; a few drops only in the eye-bath.

URTICA URENS TINCTURE diluted 1:20 in warmed water is useful for bathing and dressing burns (see the Burns section).

Index to common ailments

The ailments are listed alphabetically. Once you have selected the remedy you want from those listed under your ailment, look it up in the last section of the booklet. This section gives an alphabetical guide to many of the remedies listed and you can double check that it matches the symptoms and characteristics that you want to treat.

Remember that not all the symptoms given have to match, but the key characteristics should be represented and the general trend should be there.

Abscess (See Boils)

Altitude sickness
ARSENICUM: air hunger, anxiety, restlessness, collapse, fear of death and wanting constant reassurance.
COCA: this remedy is not included in the remedies section. It is noted for fainting fits and want of breath; headache; noises in ears; palpitations. As it is the substance used by the indigenous mountain peoples of South America, this is the one to use as a prophylactic when travelling at altitude. Sensations: Like a band across the forehead from temple to temple; pressing pain in back of head as if held from ear to ear in a vice. Shocks in head with vertigo; must lie down; often the only possible position in bed is lying on the front, on the face.

Anticipation/anxiety
ACONITE: the number one remedy for sudden and overwhelming fear of dying for whatever reason, this could be fear of war, of flying, of earthquake; claustrophobic fears; sure that death is imminent.
ARG. NIT: anticipation with claustrophobia; fear of tests; fear of appearing in public, yet these people love to appear in public. This contradiction creates tension (expansion of imagination and claustrophobia), diarrhoea and wind. They want to run away, but if they feel cornered, then they may be paralysed by anxiety and have digestive upsets. These tend to be hot blooded people, better out of doors.
GELSEMIUM: fear of up-coming events, fear of tests. These feel like impossible ordeals. Trembles, cannot speak (mouth feels as if full of tongue), chills running up and down the spine; often overwhelming fatigue; buckling at the knees.

LYCOPODIUM: extreme lack of self-confidence, yet when in their place of power they are pompous, pretentious, and their ego is inflated. 'Nice with superiors, but a tyrant at home.' Feeling of helplessness; cautious; irresolute. May shun responsibilities because of fear of not being up to the challenge.

PHOSPHORUS: anxiety before an operation, needing much reassurance. Bad reactions after anaesthetics. (See Surgery)

SILICA: apprehension and anticipation; fear of failure; bashful timidity. Delicate and refined persons who may be overly conscientious about trifling matters; great at calculation and detail. Anticipation after prolonged mental overload and consequent break-down.

Bites (Also see Stings)

APIS: stinging, itching, hot, puffy swelling. The swollen area easily indents on finger-tip pressure: when you remove your finger the area will be temporarily pale and show a small hollow or pit.

ARNICA: part feels bruised and threatens to go septic; good for horse fly bites.

LEDUM: wound feels numb and is cold, yet feels better when something cold is placed on it. This remedy has a clinically based reputation in the treatment of Lyme's disease, and should be taken as a prophylactic for tick bites when travelling in such an area. Take 30th potency twice daily for four days, then one per month while in the area.

Black eye (Also see Eye Injury)

ARNICA: take a pill of 30c or 200c immediately and there should be no local bruising.

LEDUM: when there is a mottled appearance, puffiness and the eye feels cold.

SYMPHYTUM: use when the eyeball is injured by blows, as for instance, when a toddler sticks his or her fist into it.

Boils

APIS: burning, stinging pains, swelling and redness looking like a bee sting, better with something cool on it. This remedy comes in before the boil ripens and there is pus in it. The swollen area pits on finger-tip pressure, when you remove your finger the area will be temporarily pale and indented.

ARNICA: is indicated for crops of boils all over the body, beginning with great soreness, 'don't touch me', and going on to suppuration. It can also be useful when boils will not come out, hang fire, are very sore and painful.

BELLADONNA: as with Apis, this is for the early stages: throbbing, fierce heat, bright redness and swelling; much worse from any pressure such as bandaging. The general fever picture of Belladonna will be present.

HEPAR SULPH: where there is much throbbing and sharp, sticking pains. In the early stages if given in a high potency (for instance, 200 c) it will often abort, if given low it will favour the ripening process.

LACHESIS: when the surface of the boil is very sensitive, bluish, and the central sore is surrounded by many small pimples. Often boils will occur on the left side of the body or having started there, migrate to the right side.

SILICA: for boils that occur in crops and do not heal readily, but they continue to discharge thin pus. The skin roundabout may be hardened and raised.

Bones (Also see Fractures)

ARNICA: use immediately to prevent shock and the sore bruised feeling that occurs after an accident. Touch is unbearable, even a healing hand is turned away. If an animal, then it may hide away and the injured part will be guarded.

HYPERICUM: use when fingers, toes or tail bones have been bruised or crushed and when the pains shoot up into other parts of the body.

RUTA: use for injuries to the shin bone. Use for damage to any tendons but especially the Achilles tendon.

SYMPHYTUM: do not administer until the bone has been set and then continue to give it in 6c potency, three times daily until the fracture has healed. This significantly speeds up bone formation.

Bronchitis

ACONITE: at the commencement when due to sudden chill wind or checked perspiration. The cough will be dry, hacking, and the person will be convinced that they are 'in for it'.

ANT TART: this is for serious, settled-in bronchitis. It is similar to Ipecac, but there are finer rattling sounds in the chest, and very little coughing; increased breathlessness; weakness and drowsiness; the chest seems full of mucus, but they cannot cough it up. Like Carbo Veg. this can be an important remedy for old folk with low vitality. It also may help babies and young children, when it may stop the development of pneumonia.

BELLADONNA: when there is tickling in the voice box and a dry, hacking cough, which is paroxysmal due to dryness and tightness in the upper part of the chest; worse evenings and at night. The voice box may feel sore and hot.

BRYONIA: when there is great difficulty in breathing (worse movement); a dry cough that seeming to start from the stomach, worse after a meal; stitching pains in the sides, forcing the person to hold onto, or lie on their affected side; great thirst.

CAUSTICUM: for a deep hollow, dry cough, with pain in the chest, especially under the breast-bone. Rattling in the chest when coughing and difficulty bringing up the mucus due to paralysis. Tightness of chest; must take a deep breath. Often involuntary spurting of urine when coughing.

CARBO VEG: hoarseness coming on in the evening, with rawness and scraping in the

voice box and wind-pipe, with oppression of chest. Bronchitis in old people when
there is a loose rattling in the chest on coughing or breathing. Profuse yellow, smelly,
and possibly bloody expectoration (phlegm).
IPECAC: where there is a dry spasmodic cough, ending in choking, gagging and
tickling which extends from the voice box to the lungs; rattling sounds may be heard
all over the chest. After violent paroxysms of coughing there will be retching. The face
may be pale and there will be a general shortness of breath.
LYCOPODIUM: where the smaller tubes are affected, much mucus, rattling breath;
cough and difficult, obstructed breathing; expectoration usually yellowish and thick;
right lung more affected; worse 4 to 8 p.m.
NAT. MUR: useful for chronic bronchial catarrhs, winter coughs and asthma, where
there is a profuse secretion of watery mucus.
PHOSPHORUS: dry, tickling cough, caused by irritation in the voice box; tearing
pain under the breast-bone, as if something were torn loose. Suffocative pressure
across upper part of the chest. Cough gets worse on going from warm into cold air.
Expectoration is yellowish and may be blood streaked.
SULPHUR: Chronic bronchitis where there is a large accumulation of thick mucus
looking like pus. Person has suffocative spells, oppression of the chest with burning
pains. Loud rattles may be heard all over the chest. Sulphur is a good remedy to clear
out the obstinate tail-end of bronchitis and to avoid relapse, especially in the elderly.

Burns
BURN OINTMENT: this is formulated with Calendula, Cantharis, Hypericum and
Urtica Urens (some manufacturers add a few more ingredients) and is our standard
kitchen cupboard first aid remedy for burns. Re-apply frequently.
CALENDULA & URTICA: dress burns with a diluted tincture (one part in ten of water)
or if mouth is scalded use a similar dilution as a mouthwash.
CANTHARIS: first and second degree burns – relieves the pain as if by magic.
CAUSTICUM: as Cantharis, but where burns are deeper and there is extensive
blistering, this remedy gives relief and prevents scarring. Also where the burning is
associated with paralysis and twisting of the affected limb.

Catarrh and common colds
ACONITE: when the attack comes on suddenly after exposure to dry cold winds, and
there is chilliness followed by fever; nose is dry and bunged up.
ARSENICUM: where there is a thin, watery discharge from the nose, which burns and
excoriates the upper lip, and in spite of this fluent discharge the nose feels bunged up;
the person is chilly and hugs the fire. There is a frontal headache, photophobia and
sneezing, and the sneezing does not relieve the irritation in the slightest; it is worse

going into the open air, though the burning is worse near the fire. The person is very restless and pernickety, nothings seems to be in its correct place.

CAMPHORA: it is used in the first stage, where the nose is stuffed up and the feverish symptoms of Aconite are absent. The person feels intensely chilly. There is great depression, as if all hope had been banished, with weakness and indifference. An important indicating symptom is that air breathed in feels icy cold.

CHELIDONIUM: for a loose or rattling cough.

GELSEMIUM: where there is a slowly brewing general malaise and a feeling as if flu is brewing; the head is hot and full and there is chilliness and a desire to hug the fire; the head and the eyelids droop. Colds from mild weather. There is a watery, bland discharge from the nose and much sneezing.

KALI CARBONICUM: for congestive, nasal or chesty colds with weakness.

LYCOPODIUM: here there is apt to be posterior dryness, while there is a discharge of yellowish green matter from nose. Worse 4 to 8 p.m. and worried about work.

MERCURIUS: the Mercurius discharge, though very excoriating, is not watery, but thick and it may be smelly. This person has an unsettled reaction to most things including variations in temperature, every small change upsets them.

NAT. MUR: salty watery discharges that are accompanied by blisters (cold sores) about the lips, mouth and nose; dryness at the back of the nose with loss of smell and taste. Sneezing worse in the evening while undressing and in morning on rising.

NUX VOMICA: in the first stage, when brought on by damp, cold weather, waiting for a bus, etc., associated with sneezing and a stuffed up feeling in the nose. The nose is dry; the eyes water; there is scraping in the throat, and there is dullness and oppression in the frontal region; the symptoms are worse in a warm room and better in the open air.

PULSATILLA: for a ripe cold with a thick, custard like discharge, no sneezing or excoriation, simply a thick, yellow greenish bland discharge. The person is usually not thirsty at all, and they will often be emotional and weepy.

Chicken pox

ANT. TART: spots come out very slowly. Purple discoloration around the spots, which are large and full of pus. The child is drowsy, sweaty, weak, nauseous and may develop bronchitis. A lingering state of serious ill health.

BELLADONNA: high fever with severe throbbing headache, flushed face and hot, dry skin but with cold hands and feet. Drowsy but cannot sleep. May have waking nightmares, often involving animals attacking them.

MERCURY: if the spots go septic and take on a yellow, milky hue. The spots may spread and when they burst they ooze sticky pus that then becomes crusty.

PULSATILLA: the child is weepy, cannot bear to be alone and is often thirstless.

RHUS TOX: after the fever stage is over, this is generally the main remedy, as long as no complications occur. Very itchy and restless; aching, restless legs. The spots look like a colourless jelly on a red plate.

Collapse
ARNICA: where there has been an injury and internal bleeding is suspected.
CARBO VEG: person feels icy cold to touch, may look blue or is deathly pale. Breath is very cold. Useful after loss of blood, surgery, drowning. This remedy has been called 'the corpse reviver'. Dissolve Carbo Veg. 200c tablets in water and moisten the person's lips with the solution or put dry granules on the tongue.
CAMPHORA: this remedy is not listed in the remedies section. In cases of hypothermia when the person, although feeling icy cold to the touch, throws off covers because of an aversion to heat.

Colic
CHAMOMILLA, COLOCYNTH, STAPHISAGRIA: these three remedies are to be considered when anger and/or indignation is at the root of the colic.
COLOCYNTHIS: this remedy is not listed in the remedies section. It is for a violent, agonising abdominal colic (and also useful in ovarian colic with sharp pains in the ovaries). The pains are violent, cutting, cramping making the patient twist, turn and cry out; relieved by bending double and by pressing something hard into the belly. Does not like to talk, answer, or to see anybody. Anger or chagrin is often causative.
DIOSCOREA: this remedy is not included in the remedies section. Where the pains are apt to radiate from the belly to other parts of the body, such as to the back, arms, etc. It is relieved by walking and arching the body backwards.
IPECAC: when there is griping about umbilicus as of a hand clutching; cutting pains shooting across the belly, from left to right, associated with nausea and diarrhoea.
MAGNESIA PHOSPHORICA: this remedy is not listed in the remedies section. Where there is intense and spasmodic pain, forcing the person to bend double, and accompanied by belching of gas, which does not relieve; the pains are greatly relieved by the application of warmth, such as a hot water bottle.
NUX VOMICA: for flatulent colic with desire to stool, with clutching at the anus while straining, and a sensation as if the intestines were squeezed between stones.
STAPHISAGRIA: griping pains here and there, in the whole abdomen. Swollen abdomen in children with much wind. Trapped wind. Generally excellent for the aftermath of feeling injured (perhaps after an operation), insulted, invaded and put down.

Conjunctivitis
ACONITE: eyes are red, dry and hot, as if sand is in them. Lids are swollen. Especially useful when conjunctivitis has been caused by drafts or cold wind.

APIS: eyes burn, sting, with hot, puffy swelling of lids and below eyes. Better for having something cold placed on them. This can come about as an allergic reaction to antibiotics or food.

EUPHRASIA: sticky lids, painful, hot, watery eyes, burning pain, worse in a warm room. You can also bathe the eyes with a dilute solution of tincture (one to two drops in an eye bath of boiled cooled and lightly salted water - to taste like tears).

PULSATILLA: lids stuck together. Eyes sore and red. Thick yellow discharge which does not irritate. Weepy and needy disposition.

Constipation

BRYONIA: when constipation is due to dryness of the intestinal tract and the stools are large, dry and brown, as if burnt, and are passed with great difficulty. Usually there is great thirst. They want to be alone and in a quiet environment.

CAUSTICUM: owing to a paralytic condition of the rectum the person is unable to evacuate the stool when sitting, he finds it easier to pass the stool whilst in an erect posture, almost standing.

LYCOPODIUM: has ineffectual urging to stool, but not due to irregular intestinal action, but to a constriction of the rectum, apt to be associated with haemorrhoids. It is also a useful in constipation of young children.

NAT. MUR: The stools are hard and difficult to expel, causing bleeding and smarting and soreness in the rectum. There is dryness of the rectum and the stools are crumbly in character; great weakness of the intestine.

NUX VOMICA: is of service where there is increased intestinal action, which is irregular, inharmonious and spasmodic, and this hinders rather than favours an evacuation: constant, ineffectual urging to stool, incomplete and unsatisfactory, as if a part remained behind. These people are irascible and are apt to lose their temper.

OPIUM: like Nux Vomica but with complete inactivity of the bowels, owing to muscular paralysis. Stools become impacted and are passed in little, hard, dry, black balls, and there is absolutely no urging. This state can occur after taking drugs or prescription medicine and also after surgical operations.

SEPIA: no desire or urging for days and days; the stools are hard and large; a sensation of a ball in the rectum; they cannot strain and consequently cannot expel the stool.

SILICA: when it is due to the deficient expulsive power of the rectum and spasmodic condition of the sphincter, which gives rise to the symptom that the stool slips back when partially expelled.

SULPHUR: when there is ineffectual urging to stool with a sensation of heat, fullness and discomfort in the rectum. Uneasy feeling throughout the belly; constipation alternating with diarrhoea, especially if diarrhoea drives the person out of bed. The area around the anus may be red and itchy, and the patient will scratch it.

Coughs

ACONITE: when the cough has come on suddenly after becoming chilled and is hard, dry and barking. For typical croup when there is little or no expectoration. As in all Aconite conditions, there will be fear and apprehension of death.

ANTIMONIUM TART: when the cough sounds loose, but no phlegm is raised; it seems as if every cough would raise the phlegm, but it does not. There is whistling and rattling in the chest that extends into the wind-pipe. The person may be exhausted, too weak to raise themselves up. This is a great remedy for children with threatened bronchitis, and also for older patients.

ARNICA: when the pain of continued coughing creates a 'don't touch me' state, where the person fends off help and tells the doctor to go away.

BELLADONNA: when the cough is from tickling in the voice box as from dust. It may come on in the early afternoon. It is a dry, hacking cough coming on in violent attacks with an expectoration of blood-tinged mucus. Much pain in chest.

BRYONIA: this person keeps very still because any movement aggravates them and brings on another painful bout of coughing. This is a dry, barking cough set off by irritation at the pit of the throat. While coughing the person presses their hand against their sides or chest to relieve the pain, or they hold their head because coughing brings on an explosion of head pain. The cough is worse in a warm room, and there may be a slight yellowish or blood-streaked expectoration. Usually there is thirst for infrequent but substantial amounts of water.

CAUSTICUM: where there is a tickling cough that is relieved by a sip of cold water. There is often an involuntary spurting of urine with the cough. (This symptom is also found in the cough of Natrum Muriaticum.) There is a great deal of rawness in the throat and hoarseness with eventual loss of voice.

DROSERA: when there is a maddening spasmodic cough that comes on in the evening, and every effort to raise the phlegm ends in vomiting. In whooping cough, the cough is so frequent that the person cannot catch their breath.

HEPAR SULPH: when there is a fish-bone sensation in the throat giving rise to a hoarse cough, the phlegm being loose and choking. Sudden attacks of suffocation; the child tries to speak or cry without being able to do so, grasps at throat in greatest fear, assumes a sitting posture on account of anxiety which sets in when lying down. Worse from exposure to cold air and from drinking cold water. This remedy may come in after Aconite and will often be followed by Spongia in cases of croup.

IGNATIA: when the cough is of nervous origin. It is dry, spasmodic, and comes in quick, successive shocks, at if a feather were in the throat. The more the person coughs the more they want to, and it is only stopped by an effort of the will. The cough occurs in the evening on lying down.

KALI CARBONICUM: for persistent dry, hard, night time coughs with very little expectoration which is very tenacious.

PHOSPHORUS: where there is a dry, tickling cough, which is worse from going from a warm room into the cold. It is caused by rawness in the voice box or beneath the breast bone. The cough is worse from talking, although the person is tempted to do so on account of the reassurance that company brings. This cough is worse at night and on lying down (as also are the coughs that may benefit from Silica).

SILICA: pricking as of a pin in a tonsil, sticking pains in throat, and cough when lying down with thick yellow lumpy sputum like little granules of shot, which, when broken, smell very offensive. The cough is gagging; retching worse cold drinks; worse talking, lying down and after walking. Dry and hacking cough at night, waking person from sleep. Loose cough, day and night.

SPONGIA: This remedy is not included in the remedies section. It is for a hard, croupy, ringing cough, sounding like a saw through plywood; suffocating spells, as if a cord about the neck; worse from deep breathing. The person sleeps into aggravation; worse midnight until 2 a.m.; better from warm drinks.

Cuts and abrasions

BELLIS PERENNIS: sepsis after major surgery or deep trauma.

CALENDULA: wash out the wound, bring the sides of the cut together and dress the wound with diluted tincture, using one part to ten parts water. Repeat until healed. Take a CALENDULA 30c remedy in pill form if the cut is serious. This is particularly good for healing scalp wounds. Repeat dose three times daily until healed.

HYPERCAL: this cream is ideal for cuts and grazes.

LEDUM: very useful remedy for deep puncture wounds, especially those caused by nails and/or where there may be nerve damage, swelling and risk of tetanus infection.

Dental treatment

ARNICA: pain in the tooth after a filling, or after having a tooth out. Best taken immediately after extraction, and repeated every three hours for a day or two.

CHAMOMILLA: can be used if Arnica does not work. Often the best remedy for children, who can't bear the pain and for adults of irritable temperament.

HYPERICUM: helps with nerve pain after drilling and extraction.

LEDUM: helps after an injection if the gum feels cold and is better when something cold is placed in the mouth.

MAGNESIA PHOSPHORICA: for toothache with sharp, knife-like pains that are improved by heat and rest.

NUX VOMICA: violent pain with a swollen face. Person is sensitive to everything and irritated by everyone.

Dentition

BELLADONNA: intense throbbing pain with inflammation and also for gumboils with this symptom.

CALC PHOS: this remedy is not included in the remedies section. Where the teeth are slow in their development, and where there is rapid decay of the teeth. These children may be slow learning to walk, have open fontanelles at the back of their head, and may be emaciated.

CHAMOMILLA: this tends to be the most commonly used first aid remedy for acute teething troubles where the characteristic mental state of peevishness is present; nothing distracts or relieves this child; one cheek is red, head and scalp are hot and sweaty; diarrhoea is common as an accompaniment, with stools like chopped spinach.

HEPAR SULPH: teeth exquisitely sensitive to touch. The child may feel irrational flashes of murderous anger.

MERC SOL: inflammation under a tooth; gumboil. They have bad breath and profuse saliva. Worse at night. Sensitive to any change of temperature.

PODOPHYLLUM: this remedy is not listed in the remedies section. The child bites its gums or grinds its teeth, has profuse diarrhoea which is watery, runs through the nappy, is green and smelly, it literally fills the room with stench. Worse 4 to 5 a.m.; better lying on the tummy. Diarrhoea preceded by cramping (must bend double), rumbling and gurgling, accompanied by grinding of the teeth, rolling of the head; whining and moaning during sleep, 'as if a fish were turning and tossing in a pond.' Rectal prolapse before or with the diarrhoea.

PULSATILLA: worse warm things in mouth, better out of doors. Weepy and clingy.

Diarrhoea

ACONITE: when of inflammatory origin with watery, chopped spinach, slimy and bloody stools; occurring in summer from cold drinks or checked perspiration.

ALOE: This remedy is not included in the remedies section. Stools are of jelly like mucus, they slip out without volition, there may be profound weakness; the person loses confidence in their sphincter and passes stools when they think they are passing wind. There is a sensation of weight and fullness in the pelvic region. This full feeling drives the person out of bed in morning for a stool.

ARGENTUM NITRICUM: diarrhoea following great excitement or fright. The stools are slimy and green with much flatulence, worse at night. The bowels move every time the person drinks. Should this be a child, then it appears to have but one tube extending from mouth to anus. (Gelsemium, Opium, Pulsatilla and Veratrum Alb. are also to be considered in diarrhoea from fright or disappointment.)

ARSENICUM ALBUM: vomiting and diarrhoea together with chilliness, restless anxiety and weakness. Needs someone around for reassurance, yet is not easily reassured. After bad fruit, fish or meat. Thirsty for sips of water or warm drinks. Primary characteristics are: small quantity of stool passed incessantly; burning pains; offensive odour; great weakness with anxious restlessness.

BRYONIA: in hot weather, from drinking cold water when overheated, or eating sour fruit. Wants to stay still and be quiet, and is very thirsty.

CHAMOMILLA: in teething babies. See section above.

MERCURIOUS: where the stools are slimy and bloody and accompanied by great clutching in the anus, which continues after stool, 'a never get done' sensation.

NUX VOMICA: when diarrhoea occurs after overindulgence of food/alcohol or both. The person feels worse in the morning. Stools are pappy, scanty and watery, and accompanied by ineffectual and painful urging.

OPIUM: has diarrhoea from the shutting down of the intestinal tract resulting from terrible fear or shock with insensibility of the nervous system, drowsy stupor, painlessness and general sluggishness.

PHOSPHORUS: has green mucus stools worse in the morning, often undigested and painless. The stools pass as soon as they enter the rectum; contain white particles like rice or scrapings of candle wax. Craves cold drinks that may be vomited back up within a few minutes. Wants sympathy, cuddles and reassurance that greatly improves their anxiety.

PODOPHYLLUM: (see section above for more about this remedy) spluttery, yellow and very smelly diarrhoea, painlessly passed, and with a feeling of great weakness and cramping in the belly. The diarrhoea is worse in the morning and after eating and drinking, yet there is apt to be a natural stool later on in the day. Aggravated by washing and from eating or drinking. Often a Summertime diarrhoea from eating fruit and drinking milk. Prolapsed rectum before and/or during stool.

PULSATILLA: has greenish or yellowish and changeable stools, occurring after an emotional upset or after taking mixed food the night before; eating ice cream, immediately after a meal and for children after eating party food.

SULPHUR: where the stools are changeable in colour and may contain undigested food. It occurs in the morning and drives the person out of bed; there is a great deal of abdominal uneasiness; the odour of the stool clings to the person for a long time and there is much soreness at the anus.

VERATRUM ALBUM: this remedy is not included in the remedies section. Diarrhoea and vomiting simultaneously with cold sweat, especially on forehead; collapse, cramps and coldness. Violent thirst for icy water. Worse from all fruit and vegetables and after moving the bowels.

REMEMBER THAT DIARRHOEA MAY BE UNPLEASANT AND WHEN PROLONGED CAN DEHYDRATE, BUT AS AN ACUTE, IT IS AN EFFICIENT WAY YOUR BODY HAS DEVISED TO ELIMINATE UNDESIRABLE SUBSTANCES. REMEDIES WILL RELIEVE THE DISCOMFORT AND MISERY WHILE LEAVING YOUR BODY TO HEAL ITSELF. IF THEY DO NOT RELIEVE, THEN QUICKLY SEEK PROFESSIONAL HELP.

Drugs

After taking either prescribed drugs such as antibiotics, or a mood altering substance for leisure, you may suffer from side effects. For the ill effects of hallucinogens, consult a qualified homeopath. For side effects of prescribed medicine, see below:

APIS: swellings, which itch, are hot and stinging. The pain is relieved by cold applications.

BRYONIA: does not want to move at all and is very thirsty for great drafts of water.

NUX VOMICA: angry with everyone, cannot bear contradiction. Constipation, and maybe nausea with desire to vomit, yet may be unable to do so. Very chilly. Waking 3 to 4 a.m.

SULPHUR: itching, burning skin (not swelling), much worse at night. Must scratch until skin is raw. Feeling hot. May have cystitis.

Earache

ACONITE: comes on suddenly with terror and restlessness after being out in the cold; it may start around or just after midnight.

BELLADONNA: sudden onset. Worse 3 p.m. to midnight. Redness, hot, throbbing, dilated pupils, dry flushed skin. Right ear more often affected.

CHAMOMILLA: cannot stand the pain and is extremely cross. Wants things and then throws them away. Pain worse from placing ear near warmth. Worse 9 p.m. to midnight.

FERRUM PHOS: for early stages of inflammation. Can be sweaty and thirsty. Flushed face or alternates between red and pale. Often worse at night. Flopped out.

HEPAR SULPH: stitching pain and great sensitivity to touch, drafts and cold air. Wants to be covered up. May be very irritable and abusive. Often accompanied by sore throat.

MERCURIUS: pain extends to face and teeth and is worse at night and from heat of the bed; sweaty, lots of saliva, bad breath and flabby tongue showing teeth indentations along the edge. Right ear more usually affected. Often happens in damp, changeable weather.

PULSATILLA: pains pulsating, darting and tearing. Worse from warmth, overheating and in the evening. Usually better outdoors in the fresh air. Weepy, clingy and irritable. External ear is red and swollen. May feel as if something is crawling out of the ear or as if the ears are stuffed up.

MULLEIN OIL: this remedy is not included in the remedies section. A few drops gently warmed should be put into the painful ear to ease the pain and help to cure the condition. This may be used together with the indicated remedy.

Eye injury (Also see Black Eye)
ACONITE: if eye has a piece of grit in it, or if the socket has been injured. Acute pain, flowing tears, redness and huge distress.
SYMPHYTUM: use when the eyeball is injured by blows, or when a toddler sticks his or her fist into it.
See 'Eye Strain'.

Eye inflammation and eye strain
EUPHRASIA: 'Pink Eye' with profuse tears that are acrid and burning.
RUTA: good for eyestrain from prolonged use and/or in poor light, where eyes are red, sore, hot and painful. Use when the eyeball is injured by blows (cf. Symphytum).

Fainting
ACONITE: from shock or violent emotions or panic/terror. Unaccountable fear.
IGNATIA: from hearing bad news, from grief, from seeing blood, or from being in a crowded room.
PULSATILLA: from a hot stuffy atmosphere.

Fever (Also see Common Sense Measures)
ACONITE: in intense fevers of fast onset, with chilliness on the slightest movement; dry heat of skin, thirst, red cheeks, quickened respiration; full, bounding, rapid, tense pulse, with mental anxiety, fear of dying and aggravation towards evening.
BELLADONNA: when, like Aconite, the onset is rapid and there are symptoms of delirium leading to hallucinations with dilated pupils and a hot head; bounding pulse and sensations of throbbing. Marked aggravation around 3 in the afternoon; diminished thirst, even repugnance of water.
BRYONIA: when the fever is accompanied by a hard, tense pulse, intense headache, dry mouth, tongue coated white down the middle; person avoids light and motion. Thirst for large quantities of water at long intervals.
FERRUM PHOS: in the early stages of fevers, it stands midway between the activity of Acon. and Bell. and the sluggishness and torpidity of Gels. When there is a flushed face; red eyes; restlessness. Great nervousness at night: desires to get out of bed, and wishes to run around, but is so weak that he falls over; very talkative and find situations hilarious.
GELSEMIUM: where the fever has crept up gradually, and now there is aching, alternating fever and chills, and overwhelming weariness; drowsiness, dullness and dizziness; soreness of muscles and absence of thirst; great prostration and symptoms which return.
PHOSPHORUS: is similar to Ferrum Phos. to start with (see above), but then develops

into a stupefied fever, characterised by sleepiness, which becomes worse at twilight and may then be accompanied by many fears.
PULSATILLA: a changeable state where chilliness predominates; fever without thirst, with oppression and sleepiness; worse about 2 or 3 in the afternoon.

Flu

The homeopathic remedy INFLUENZINUM 200c can be used as a preventative. It can be taken once a month during the flu season and more often if contact is made with someone suffering from the flu. Many homeopathic pharmacies make it fresh from that year's flu vaccine. Some homeopaths say that it is more effective than the conventional flu shot and without any side effects. Studies in England and India between 1968 and 1970 using homeopathic Influenzinum as a preventative showed that this remedy was highly effective at preventing the flu.

ACONITE: Flu with great restlessness and fear of death. This remedy is useful if the flu symptoms came on very suddenly, especially after exposure to a dry, cold wind, or from an emotional shock or fright. They are worse in a warm room, in the evening and at night.
ARSENICUM: aching, thirsty for sips of warm drinks. Burning pains here and there. Extreme weakness yet they are restless. Extremely chilly. Worse after midnight. Wants to be with a friend to calm their many fears.
BAPTISIA: this remedy is not listed in the remedies section. Flu with high fever and a feeling of being bruised all over. This remedy is useful for flu that comes on suddenly and the individual feels bruised and sore all over (like Arnica), the body and limbs feel as if they are all in bits and scattered about. There is profuse sweating with a high fever and an intense thirst. The face is dull red in colour and people who need this remedy look dazed and sluggish as if they may fall asleep at any time. This remedy is also for gastric flu with vomiting and diarrhoea.
BELLADONNA: This remedy is useful when a very high fever comes on suddenly usually as a result of exposure to infection or from the head getting cold, wet, or they have become overheated. The face is flushed and bright red, the throat is sore, the eyes are wide and staring and the pupils dilated, there is possible confusion and delirium. The individual feels better when they stand or sit upright and in a warm room. They are worse from any noise or bright light or movement. They are worse from lying down and at night and symptoms tend to affect the right side of their body.
BRYONIA: Flu with a severe, throbbing headache, wants to be left alone. This remedy is useful for a flu that comes on slowly, they ache all over and the remedy tends to be characterised by a violent headache that is made worse by coughing or by even slightly moving the eyes. The headache feels better if firm pressure is applied and

they can sleep. There is dehydration and a need to drink lots of fluids at infrequent intervals. They feel very irritable, and want to be left alone and at home. They may be worrying about financial problems. They feel worse from any excitement, noise, touch, movement or bright light, from eating and coughing and at around 3 a.m. and 9 p.m.

EUPATORIUM PERFOLIATUM: flu with bone pains so severe that it actually feels as if the bones were broken. The muscles ache and feel sore and bruised. The individual moans and groans and everything hurts. They feel worse for any kind of movement. They have a bursting headache and sore eyes. There is a lot of sneezing, the nose is runny, the chest is sore and coughing makes the head hurt. These people want ice-cold water although it brings on violent chills in the small of the back. Chill between 7 to 9 a.m. They don't sweat much but when they do they feel better except for their head.

GELSEMIUM: Flu with chills and paralytic weakness. This tends to be the number one flu remedy. In contrast to Aconite, Baptisia and Belladonna the symptoms of Gelsemium come on slowly after exposure to infection or as a result of worrying about a forthcoming task. There is a sore throat and chills, which run up and down the spine. They may have a splitting headache, which is better after urinating. There is a general feeling of fatigue, the legs feel weak and shaky and they just want to lie in bed. The eyelids are droopy, the head feels heavy and they may have double vision. There is pain felt in the bones. Although they may have a fever they do not sweat and they are not thirsty. They feel better in the fresh air, when moving around and bending forward. They feel worse in the early morning and last thing at night, in the sun, when exposed to tobacco smoke.

FLU WILL USUALLY RUN ITS COURSE IN A FEW DAYS. A REMEDY WILL HELP YOU RECOVER QUICKLY SO THE WEAKNESS DOES NOT CONTINUE FOR DAYS AFTER.

Fractures and injuries of joints

ARNICA: best repeated hourly for the first 24 hours until the shock is over. Fractures should be set by a qualified doctor as soon as swelling has subsided. Arnica will help to ensure that this occurs rapidly.

BELLIS PERENNIS: very useful for falls on the tailbone, (also look at Hypericum) abdominal injuries and for sprains with bruising and soreness. Bellis also has an important affinity with the breast and is useful after a blow to the breast.

BRYONIA: the pain is much, much worse whenever the affected part is moved, so they will often hold onto the painful part to keep it still.

CALC. PHOS: for use when bones will not mend, when Symphytum fails to act.

LEDUM: should follow ARNICA if the bruising remains and turns yellow.

RHUS TOX: when the person feels worse at night and from the cold and wet. They just cannot get comfortable and are restless.

RUTA: use for damage to tendons, especially the Achilles tendon, wrist, ankle, and any joints where sensation is one of constriction of movement. Good for RSI (Repetitive Strain Injury). Use when the eyeball is injured by blows. Good for eyestrain from prolonged use.

SYMPHYTUM: do not administer until bone has been set and then continue to give it in 6c potency, three times daily until the fracture has healed. The use of this remedy significantly speeds up
bone formation.

Grief (Also see Shock)

IGNATIA: for bereavement and after miscarriage or abortion with private grief with hidden tears. Whatever the cause, their emotional outbursts are quickly controlled: short sobs, involuntary sighing, constant swallowing, bites inside of cheek... The sensation in the heart and chest area is of constriction and pressure as of a heavy weight. This response to grief is similar to Natrum Mur. which presents with chronic withheld grief and brooding sorrow.

Hay fever

ALLIUM CEPA: this remedy that is prepared from the onion is not listed in the remedies section. The hay fever begins with frequent sneezing. Watery discharge drips from the nose which feels raw; it burns the lip and wings of nose; it leaves red streaks as it flows over the skin (cf. Arsenicum). At the same time the eyes water profusely, but do not sting or become inflamed. (Reverse of Euphrasia). Generally begins on the left side and goes to right; on rising from bed; very sensitive to odour of flowers and the skin of peaches.

ARSENICUM ALBUM: nasal discharge burns a red streak over upper lip and about the wings of the nose. The sneezing is relentless accompanied by profuse, watery and burning nasal discharge. The typical Arsenicum person is anxious, restless, often asthmatic, and their worst hour is soon after midnight. The sneezing is no joke! It starts from tickling in one spot in the nose. After sneezing there is no relief because the tickling is just as bad as before.

CARBO VEG: frequent sneezing, with constant violent crawling and tickling in the nose; tears and biting pain in and above the nose. Ineffectual desire to sneeze with crawling sensation in the left nostril. Watery discharge and sneezing day and night. Suffers from heat; is chilled by cold; sweats in a hot room. No comfortable place.

EUPHRASIA: this remedy is not listed in the remedies section, but has a mention in the eye inflammation section. Sneezing with profuse acrid tears, red eyes, plus profuse bland nasal discharge (reverse of Allium Cepa). It is the eyes that bear the brunt of this species of hay fever. Eyes worse open air and wind.

GELSEMIUM: sneezing; hot face; feeling of great weight and tiredness in whole body and limbs. Violent morning paroxysms of sneezing from tingling in the nose. Watery, burning discharge. Curious symptom is a feeling from throat up to left nostril, like a stream of scalding water.

LACHESIS: paroxysms of sneezing worse after sleep even in the day time. Headache extending into nose, with frequent and violent paroxysms of sneezing. Mucous membrane of the nose is inflamed and thickened. There is a dry stuffed sensation throughout the head. The face is red and puffy; eyes seem almost pressed out. Red, sore nostrils and lips; throat sensitive to touch or pressure.

NAT. MUR: squirming as from a small worm in the nose. Watery discharge from eyes and nose. Profuse discharge, has to lay a towel under the nose. Wakes with headache; after rising nasal discharge with violent and frequent sneezing. Loss of taste and smell; cough from tickling in throat pit. Tears burn and the corners of the eyes are red and sore. Characteristics: Worse in sun; desire for salt in hay fever, better at seaside, may even be cured by a swim in the sea.

NUX VOMICA: distressing prolonged paroxysms of sneezing. Excessive irritation in nose, eyes and face. Heat as if a hot radiator were near it. Itching extends to voice box and down the wind pipe. Very irritable; very sensitive to cold.

SABADILLA: this remedy is not listed in the remedies section. (As Euphrasia is to the eyes, so Sabadilla is to the nose.) Violent sneezing with copious watery discharge from the nose, but the nostrils are stuffed up; breathing through the nose is laboured; snoring. Itching in nose; bleeding from nose; severe frontal pains. There may also be redness of eyelids. Very sensitive to the smell of garlic.

SILICA: begins with itching and tingling in the nose. Violent sneezing and burning discharge. Itching right at the back of the mouth at the orifice of the eustachian tubes.

Headache

ARNICA: when the cause is injury.

ARG. NIT: where there is a sensation as if the head were enlarged, and the headache is accompanied with dizziness. The pains increase to such a degree that the person almost loses their senses, but pressure from wrapping the head up relieves. Like Pulsatilla they may feel hot and are better for fresh air and wide-open spaces.

BELLADONNA: where the pain is worse on the right side and worse in the frontal region and is aggravated by lying down. There is much throbbing, reaching a crescendo of stabbing, sharp pain, driving the patient almost wild. They are greatly aggravated by light, noise or jarring. Usually the face is red and the pupils are dilated.

BRYONIA: splitting frontal headache extending backward and down the neck, shoulders and the back. It is worse in the morning and is aggravated by any motion, even of the eyeballs. Infrequent thirst for large quantities of water.

CHINA: headache with violent throbbing of the arteries in the neck; head feels as though the skull would burst; sensation as if the brain beat in waves against the skull. Headache from blood loss.

GELSEMIUM: dull, heavy ache with droopy eyelids, and soreness of the eyeballs when moving them. Dim or double vision. Pulsating pain in forehead and eyeballs. Never well since the flu. The headache commences in the nape, passes over the head and settles in an eye; worse in the morning; relieved by a discharge of urine. The face is dark red and looks bewildered; the person is listless and appears as if under the influence of alcohol; there is also a feeling of a band around the head.

IGNATIA: where there is heaviness in the head as if congested, relieved by stooping. There is a pain as if a nail were driven into the side or the back of the head; there may be much sighing; the headache ends in vomiting or in a copious discharge of pale urine. It is greatly aggravated by smoking or smelling tobacco. It is of a hysterical origin, coming on after anger or disappointment – where an ideal has been smashed.

KALI CARBONICUM: congestive headache with stitching or throbbing pain.

KALI PHOSPHORICUM: pains are stitching, sudden and sharp. Pain in the back of head, better for rising/standing up.

NAT. MUR: has a headache as from the beating of little hammers in the head that is worse from moving the head or eyeballs. Vision may be affected with zigzag and peripheral disturbances. Worse reading; worse motion, even of eyes; worse light; worse noise; worse reading; worse light and sun; worse menses; aggravated 10 a.m. to 3 p.m; better lying in a dark room; better pressure on eyes.

NUX VOMICA: is a headache due to gastric troubles, usually due to carousing and drinking, and it occurs in the morning. The headache is either at the back of the head or over one or the other eye, and is often associated with vomiting of food and violent retching. It is often associated with constipation and possibly piles. These people are easily angered and consolation is viewed as interference and annoys them.

PULSATILLA: this headache is congestive, mostly frontal or above the eyes; worse by warmth and mental exertion, and worse in the evening, better out of doors and for fresh breezes. There may be wandering pains, from one part of the head to another. Gastric, rheumatic or uterine symptoms often accompany the headache. Pulsatilla people are almost always better for consolation and cuddles.

PHYTOLACCA: headache is accompanied by backache and a generally sore, bruised feeling.

SEPIA: headache from over-care, housework, exhaustion. There may be a sharp pain in the lower part of the brain that shoots upward. Heaviness of eyelids during the headache. Left-sided headache, above left eye; blurred vision before headache; drooping of eyelids during headache. They cannot bear light, noise, company or consolation. It may be accompanied by uterine discharges and often by nausea and vomiting. The headache is relieved by either sleep or violent motion, such as dancing. SILICA: this headache is of a nervous origin, and may be caused by excessive mental exertion. The pains come up from back of the neck, over the top of the head, and so down upon the forehead, settling over one eye, usually the right eye; worse from draft of air, a cold room, from noise, motion or jarring; better from wrapping the head up warmly, and (like Gelsemium) from urination.

STAPHISAGRIA: sensation of an immovable ball or dullness in the forehead and of emptiness at the back of the head. Pain on stooping as if the head would burst, as if the back of the head were compressed, internally and externally, as if the brain were not large enough for the space. Violent yawning (often followed by involuntary tears) after the headache.

Head injury

ARNICA: this is the one to use immediately. If sleepiness follows, DIAL 999, call your doctor, or go to 'Accident and Emergency'. Contact a homeopath for subsequent treatment.

NATRUM SULPH: this remedy is not listed in the remedies section. When the person is confused or feels depressed after a head injury. Also convulsions after head injury. Contact a homeopath for subsequent treatment.

OPIUM: Head injury, concussion with somnolence and confusion. Cerebral accident with stupor, bloated and mottled face, great heat and perspiration, snoring respiration, constricted pupils.

Injuries (See Fractures)

Measles

ACONITE: high fever and catarrh before the typical rash comes out. Red eyes; dry barking cough; itching burning skin; rash like little grains of corn. Tossing about and very frightened.

BELLADONNA: bright red rash, skin very hot; dilated pupils; sore throat and no thirst. Temperature may be alarmingly high, yet often the feet and hands are icy cold. There may be hallucinations, typically of being chased by monsters and wild animals.

GELSEMIUM: drowsy and flopped-out state; heavy eyelids, red eyes; burning runny nose; sore throat; sneezing; severe headache at the back of the head. Feels alternately hot and cold.

PULSATILLA: a common remedy for measles once the rash is out. Thick catarrh, usually yellow to green in colour; eyes water and lids stick together. Dry mouth and no thirst. Cough dry at night and looser during the day. If there is a very high temperature then this is unlikely to be the right remedy, try Belladonna.

Menses

ACONITE: late/scanty after a fright or becoming chilled.

BELLADONNA: Hot heavy blood loss.

CAULOPHYLLUM: for premenstrual lower back pain. Characteristically there are aching, sore limbs pre-menstrually

CIMICIFUGA: for intolerably painful menstrual cramps and also for suppressed menses from emotional causes.

IPECAC: Nausea before and during period.

KALI PHOS: for severe menstrual and pre-menstrual headaches.

MAGNESIA PHOSPHORICA: for sharp menstrual cramps when heat and bending over ameliorates the pain.

PULSATILLA: Period late, with wandering pains and changing stmptoms.

Motion sickness

COCCULUS: feels as if intoxicated with stupefaction of the head and numbness and unsteadiness of limbs. Feels worse for moving about or looking at a moving object. Headache, dizziness, sweating, saliva and exhaustion. Better lying down.

IPECAC: there is a constant desire to vomit, yet they do not feel the slightest relief from vomiting. They have a clean tongue. They need to be out in fresh air.

NUX VOMICA: great sensitivity to least movement or noise, constant nausea, very chilly, splitting headache, buzzing in ears.

TABACUM: this remedy is not included in the remedies section. Icy coldness and sweat, pallor and nausea with dizziness.

Mumps

APIS: swelling is soft, puffy, rosy looking and tender, like a bee sting. The child is not thirsty and cannot bear becoming heated.

BELLADONNA: glowing red face which is often swollen only on the right side. Violent shooting pains. The child is sensitive to cold and may have cold feet and hands although the head and torso are burning hot. There may be hallucinations, typically of being chased by wild animals.

BRYONIA: hard swelling with great tenderness. Child is irritable with dry, possibly cracked lips. Slightest motion is painful, therefore the child lies as still as possible, not moving a muscle, except when needing to quench a thirst for large and frequent drinks of water.

MERCURY: breath offensive; saliva increased, leaving a dribble patch on the pillow; sweaty and uncomfortable. Thirsty for cool drinks. Swelling is usually on the right side. There may have been nightmares of fighting and pursuit.

RHUS TOX: face and neck swollen on the left side. Child feels worse at night and from the cold and wet; they may have cold sores. Usually cannot get comfortable

and is restless.
PULSATILLA: use if the child is weepy and clinging, and immediately should the swelling move to the breasts or testicles.

Nausea and vomiting (Also see Common Sense Measures)
ARSENICUM: vomiting from spoiled food. See 'Diarrhoea' above.
CAULOPHYLLUM: for pre-menstrual and pregnancy nausea.
IPECAC: tongue is clean and there is constant queasiness, yet they do not feel the slightest relief from vomiting. They are neither thirsty nor hungry. They may want to be outdoors. Can be due to motion or the after effects of hot sun or overeating.
NUX VOMICA: wants to vomit but cannot. Chilly and intensely irritable.
PHOSPHORUS: great thirst for water, iced drinks, ice-cream but vomits them up shortly afterwards. Feels better in company.

Pregnancy and childbirth
CAULOPHYLLUM: for strengthening uterine contractions during labour, for expelling a partially-retained placenta and for severe afterbirth pains which fly in all directions. Also for pregnancy nausea.
CIMICIFUGA: for dilating a rigid cervix during labour. Intolerable after-birth pains experienced in groins. Contractions move from side to side.
KALI CARBONICUM: for severe lower back pain during labour. Nagging pain in back, buttocks and thighs.
KALI PHOS: for weak ineffectual contractions during labour. Often recommended for exhaustion. Helpful during labour if there are no symptoms.
PHYTOLACCA: for breastfeeding problems such as sore or cracked nipples, mastitis, blocked milk ducts and over-production of milk. Pains intense; radiate out from around the nipple.
PULSATILLA: weepiness, clinginess, and pleading for help. Cantractions short and weak or stop completely. Worse in a stuffy room.
SECALE: Like Pulsatilla intolerant to stuffy rooms but emotionally more stupefied in labour with much longer contractions. If these stop trembling may start. Can be used to antidote the ill effects of Syntometrine. Also useful in aiding the expulsion of a retained placenta.
SEPIA: Pains severe, dragging down, much relieved by exercise. Emotionally irritable or indifferent to love ones, responds badly to sympathy. Sluggish and weepy.

Shock (Also see Fainting and Grief)
ACONITE: if the person is agitated, restless or fearful after a car accident, violence, or earthquake then this is the remedy. Usually there will be an overwhelming fear of dying.

ARNICA: this remedy should be given as soon as possible after a physical injury where there is bruising whether external or internal.
BACH FLOWER RESCUE REMEDY: this remedy is not included in the remedies section. As the name implies, this is good to use after any trauma and can be purchased from most health food shops.

Sore throat

ACONITE: burning, bright red, acute inflammation, often occurring at night after exposure to cold winds. Cannot swallow, yet thirst for cold water.
BELLADONNA: an acute picture similar to ACONITE, but with aversion to drinking. The right side of the throat is usually affected first. Tonsils enlarged, throat feels constricted, difficult swallowing, yet constant desire for empty swallowing which brings on choking and spasms. The fever is often accompanied by dilated pupils and redness of face. The tongue is bright red and can look like a strawberry.
HEPAR SULPH: when the throat is extremely sensitive to touch outside, while inside it feels full of splinters or as if a fish bone were stuck there. This person cannot tolerate the least cold, even an arm out of bedcovers intensifies the pain unbearably.
KALI CARBONICUM: hoarseness, loss of voice, difficulty swallowing with gagging and vomiting and a sensation of a fish bone stuck in throat.
LACHESIS: for left-sided quinsy, extending to right side; worse warm drinks, better cold drinks. Purple or bluish discoloration. Choking from clothing around neck, from slight pressure or touch.
MERCURIUS: Painful dryness of throat with pain on swallowing, but is constantly obliged to swallow the profuse watery saliva that gathers in their mouth. Tongue is swollen and bears the imprint of teeth along its edge. Whitish, smeary lumps and pus on the tonsils, with sharp sticking pain on swallowing. Painfully hawks up large lumps from the throat. This person cannot tolerate even small temperature changes.
PHYTOLACCA: Best used when the throat is dark or bluish-red, feels full, as if choked. Swallowing sends pain up into ears, if severe cannot swallow at all. Painfully stiff neck and shoulders.

Sprains & strains

BEFORE YOU CALL THE DOCTOR - GIVE ARNICA! This is excellent for getting rid of the bruised, sore feeling that comes from too much physical effort, for aching muscles and joints. The part feels sore and is painful if moved. Arnica oil or ointment can be rubbed on the painful part unless the skin is broken.
BRYONIA: the pain is much, much worse for the slightest movement, so the person will often hold on to it to keep it still.
LEDUM: for sprained wrist/ankle if it feels better with a cold application. Can be used when the injury swells and turns puffy, blue, cold and feels numb.

Get Well Soon

Stings

Lemon juice or vinegar helps ease the pain of a wasp sting and a solution of bicarbonate of soda or soap will help relieve bee stings. Everyone knows about dock leaves relieving nettle stings, they are also effective for insect stings!

APIS: for severe reactions to bee/wasp/jelly fish stings, where there are red and puffy, hot, tense swellings and burning, stinging pains. Also for severe allergic reactions to antibiotics and other drugs*

ARNICA TINCTURE: very helpful when applied immediately; especially good for bee and wasp stings and horse fly bites.

CANTHARIS: for severe reaction to stings where the part is swollen, red and burning, as if scalded. If this progresses then think of Lachesis.

LACHESIS: Bites that go septic and turn a bluish, purplish colour. Blue-black swellings. Skin around bites is yellow, green, lead-coloured, bluish red or black. Intense itching, almost driving to distraction, also burning pains, mostly at night, but also by paroxysms in daytime. Least touch or pressure produces black and blue spots.

LEDUM: the part feels cold, is painful to touch and feels better if something cool is pressed on it.

LEDUM TINCTURE: especially good for midges and mosquitoes when applied immediately.

STAPHISAGRIA: a great relief after midge and mosquito attack, where a sense of being harassed with a feeling of indignation (how dare they) and itching persist.

*In the case of a severe allergic reaction, such as anaphylactic shock, hospital treatment must be sought immediately (or the patient's own EpiPen used instantly) but you can also try a remedy at the same time, If the remedy is homeopathic to the case, improvement will ensue, and you can repeat that remedy until a stable state has been established, and if not, you have not wasted precious time, and medical intervention will be at hand.

Sunburn

CANTHARIS, BURN OR URTICA OINTMENT, ALSO URTICA TINCTURE, ten drops in half a cup of cooled boiled water will soothe if sponged on the skin.

Sunstroke

BELLADONNA: burning hot, dry skin, throbbing headache that is worse lying down. Dilated pupils.

BRYONIA: splitting headache with nausea that gets worse every time the person moves. This requires them to remain perfectly still.

GELSEMIUM: bursting sensation in head and eyeballs, or feels as though there is a band around the head. Weak, trembling, dazed and dizzy.

GLONOINE: this remedy is not listed in the remedies section. The pains are more severe than those of Belladonna. Face may be dusky, purple and puffy. Pain worse bending head backwards. It is better uncovering and for open air.

NATRUM CARB: this remedy is not listed in the remedies section. It is of service in acute and chronic effects of sunstroke. Unconsciousness. In chronic cases debility, anaemia and weakness; inability to think or to perform any mental work; dizziness; feels stupefied if he tries to exert himself.

GIVE ONE OF THESE REMEDIES IN 30c POTENCY EVERY 15 - 30 MINUTES UNTIL THE PERSON IMPROVES.

Surgery

Homeopathy can help with pre-operation nerves and with the bleeding or pain that may follow. Also helps with the after effects of anaesthesia.

ARNICA: should be taken immediately before the operation and also for 3 to 4 days afterwards to promote healing and to prevent bleeding. Amazing pain relief!

HYPERICUM: use if nerves are damaged. There may be shooting pains which could point to the beginning of an infection.

PHOSPHORUS: for the spaced out feeling after a general anaesthetic, also nausea. Also good for pre-operation nerves.

STAPHISAGRIA: generally excellent for the aftermath of deep surgery and if the scar hurts. A must after catheterisation, abortion/termination (cf. Ignatia) and where sphincters have been dilated. Good for the feeling of having being misused and invaded.

SYMPHYTUM: for phantom limb pains post-amputation.

Teething/toothache (see Dentition)

Urinary disorders

APIS: urine is scanty or suppressed, with general puffiness and drowsiness, lack of thirst and suffocative sensation on lying down.

BELLADONNA: Involuntary urination during sleep in children. Sensations of turning and twisting motion in bladder as of a worm. Spasmodic, crampy straining; stinging, burning, from region of kidneys to bladder. Shooting in bladder when moving. Acute urinary infections. Urine scanty, dark and turbid like yeast.

CANTHARIS: persistent and violent urging to urinate, with violent gripping pains; the urine is passed only in drops, and scalds when passing through the urethra; intense burning on urination, and aching in the small of the back.

CAUSTICUM: paralysis of the bladder; involuntary urination while coughing.

EQUISETUM: This remedy is not included in the remedies section. Involuntary urination, dribbling with marked irritation, painful urination and urging; bladder sore and tender; great desire to pass water from pressure on the bladder; frequent painful urging with either excessive or scanty flow of urine, which is high coloured and contains mucus; there is also aching in the region of the kidneys.

LYCOPODIUM: here the urine is turbid and bad smelling and deposits a red sand; child cries before passing water on account of crystals in the urine, the nappy is stained yellow.

NAT. MUR: Nocturnal urination, especially during first part of sleep. The urine is colourless and profuse. In general the person whether child or adult, will display the mental characteristics typical of this remedy.

NUX VOMICA: where there are painful, ineffectual efforts to pass urine, with scanty discharge and burning; dribbling of urine in old people from enlarged prostate. Spasms of the bladder; frequent calls; little and often.

OPIUM: retention of urine from fright and after operations or hospitalised childbirth.

SEPIA: irritable bladder, involuntary escape of urine during first sleep. Red sediment in the urine which is acid and smelly. There will be an accompanying sensation of weight and heaviness in the pelvic area.

STAPHISAGRIA: cystitis after sexual intercourse, or after catheterisation, with cutting and burning right up into the kidneys every time urine is passed, which is even worse afterwards. Urging to urinate, yet scarcely a spoonful is passed, mostly of a dark-yellow colour; at times dribbling of urine, always followed by a sensation as if the bladder were not yet empty.

PULSATILLA: frequent urging to urinate, as if the bladder is too full; urine turbid. A useful remedy during pregnancy.

Vomiting and diarrhoea

ARSENICUM: this is the number one prescription for food poisoning with vomiting and diarrhoea occurring together. Sudden sinking of strength; worse at night; much tossing and turning; overwhelming weakness and fear of imminent death; violent burning pains. You can use this with confidence for babies displaying vomiting and diarrhoea with restlessness, as well as those suffering from 'Delhi-belly'.

VERATRUM ALBUM: this remedy is not included in the remedies section. Symptoms are similar to Arsenicum but there is less restlessness. In addition there is great coldness of the skin and clammy sweat, especially on the forehead. Cold feeling in blood vessels and bones. Craving for acid fruit, salty things and cold drinks. Intense thirst. Sudden sinking of strength with stomach spasms and leg cramps. Worse before menses; worse in the Spring and Autumn. Veratrum Album and Arsenicum are the main remedies where vomiting and watery diarrhoea occur simultaneously.

Whooping cough (Also see Cough Section)

ARNICA: if the child cries before or after a paroxysm of violent coughing, then Arnica often sooths away the pain. It's a good palliative remedy.

BRYONIA: the cough is dry and is worse after eating or drinking. Increased thirst is common yet drinking may cause vomiting. The pain of coughing may make the child jump out of bed and the child may clutch its sides from the pain.

CARBO VEG: burning pains in chest, cold sweat, cold pinched face, spasmodic hollow dry cough. Violent coughing fits bringing up a little yellow or bloody phlegm or followed by retching and gagging.

DROSERA: worse lying down, after midnight and after drinking. Barking cough due to crawling, tickling in the throat. Pain in chest such that the breath is kept back when speaking or coughing. Pain just below the ribs, in the pit of the stomach from coughing. Choking for breath because the paroxysms of coughing follow each other so fast. Cough followed by vomiting. If you enquire how the 'victim' feels you may hear that they literally feel stuck and trapped in the coughing fits.

IPECAC: child stiffens, loses breath, goes pale, relaxes and vomits mucus. Feels sick all the time. May bleed through the nose or mouth.

MAG. PHOS: this remedy is not included in the remedies section. True spasmodic cough with contraction of fingers and staring, open eyes, coming on in paroxysms from dry, tickling in the throat, without expectoration. General improvement from cuddling a hot water bottle. Whooping cough is worse at night and accompanied with difficulty in lying down.

IF YOUR CHILD HAS BEEN INOCULATED (AS MOST HAVE) OR HAS SUCH LOW VITALITY THAT HE OR SHE PRODUCES LOW GRADE WHOOPING COUGH SYMPTOMS THEN CARBO VEG. CAN BE THE ONE TO TRY. IN OTHER WORDS, IF ALL OF THE ABOVE DESCRIPTIONS OF WHOOPING COUGH ARE UNCLEAR AND THE SYMPTOMS CONFUSED, YOU MAY BEGIN BY GIVING ONE OR TWO DOSES OF CARBO VEG. 30C AFTER WHICH, SHOULD IMPROVEMENT NOT BE MAINTAINED ON GIVING FURTHER DOSES, ONE OF THE ABOVE REMEDIES MAY BE INDICATED. CARBO VEG. HAS THE CAPACITY TO 'WAKE UP' YOUR CHILD'S RESPONSES TO THE DISEASE AND BRING OUT A CLEARER PICTURE UPON WHICH TO PRESCRIBE.

Remedies

In this section you will find more detailed information about 50 commonly used remedies. The remedies are listed alphabetically. When looking for a remedy that fits the symptoms presented by the patient look at the whole picture, not only at the physical symptoms, but also at the mental and emotional state of the person, what the circumstances are surrounding the ailment, and what makes it better or worse.

Of the 50 remedies you will notice 9 are indicated as constitutional as well as acute remedies. In certain respects the differentiation into remedies that are used constitutionally or for acute work is arbitrary, as an indicated remedy may be used for either. However, it follows from clinical experience, that certain types fall into certain categories, hence a differentiation can be made. You will understand 'the why of it' as you begin to read the following remedy pictures. In these descriptions we are putting our focus upon their use during childhood and adolescent. Obviously the symptoms do not only fit one stage in life and can be transposed to all stages.

If you find you are repeatedly prescribing the same remedy for someone then it may be that a constitutional remedy needs to be given for the underlying chronic condition, as it this state that is driving the acute flare-up for which you are prescribing. In other words your remedy is acting superficially, and not curing the whole illness. However, unless the underlying state is really clear and happens to fit one of the given remedy pictures, prescribing at the constitutional level is a detailed process and should be left to an experienced proffesional homeopath.

If you happen to see a clear constitutional picture that obviously fits one of the remedies described here and you feel confident enough to have ago, we suggest that you give two doses of 200c, one at night and the other the following morning. When prescribing constitutionally you cannot do any harm so long as you 'watch and wait'. It is impatience that could lead you astray. We suggest that you give it a month before coming to a definite conclusion as to whether a remedy has acted or not. Please do not be tempted to try out many remedies at short intervals, as each prescription may be having long-term effects of which you may be unaware. The worst that can happen if you follow the watch and wait dictum is that the remedy may have no effect whatsoever in which case the underlying disease will continue unchanged.

Aconite

These people, often babies and children, appear frightened, they toss about and the bedclothes may be thrown off. They may express a fear of dying, or the fears may be unaccountable, with palpitations and tingling sensations throughout the body. Inflammation may be anywhere. Face red, flushed, swollen; on rising the face becomes deathly pale, or one cheek is red, the other pale. Pulse hard, quick, full. These symptoms come on suddenly, as if out of nowhere and are violent and frightening. The pains are intolerable, driving the person crazy; they may shriek with the pain. Internal pains are burning, while outer parts may feel numb, enlarged, or they burn, tingle, prickle or crawl. There may be burning thirst with the high, dry fever. The person feels generally better once perspiration starts.

If restlessness, heat and redness are observed, ask yourself or the person if they have been out in the cold, especially on a windy day, or have recently had a fright of some kind. This remedy has gained laurels in the nursery as well as in disaster situations such as after earthquakes. There may be a desire for cold water or bitter drinks.

Worse: From being out in the cold; midnight; tobacco smoke; light and noise.
Better: Open air; rest.

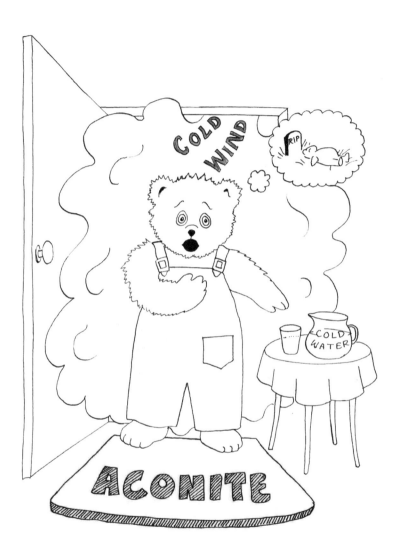

Antimonium Tartaricum
For respiratory problems with increased secretion of mucus, but scanty expectoration, with rattling in the wind-pipe and suffocative shortness of breath, alternating with a loose, coarse, rattling cough. The chest seems full of mucus, yet less and less is raised. The cough is often followed by vomiting or sleep. Nausea comes in waves with great weakness and cold sweat, loathing or anxiety. Sinking strength. Also for pustular skin eruptions, such as occur in chicken pox (cf. Mercurius & Rhus Toxicendron).

Worse: Lying down; in cold; damp weather; in the evening and at night; being looked at; wants to be left alone.
Better: Sitting up; from expectoration; sour drinks.

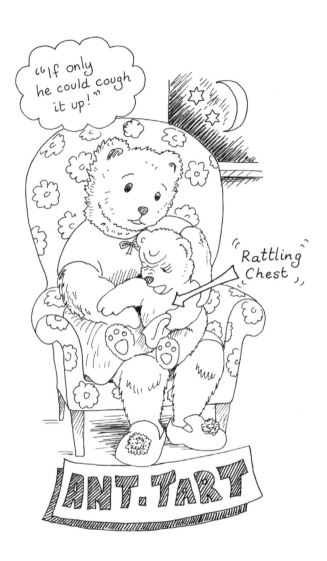

Apis

Bee stings, or any swelling which has this look about it, of red, rosy, puffy skin under tension. Also for kidney pain, swollen glands, tonsillitis and mumps. The person will be thirstless and complain of stinging, burning pains with restlessness and an aversion to being touched. They cannot bear heat and need fresh air. A state may arise which is dazed, almost stupefied, in which movements are clumsy. Later, in severe cases with brain inflammation, there may be shrieking, boring the head into the pillow and screaming.

Worse: All heat/hot drinks/baths; right side; late afternoon; after sleeping.
Better: Open air; cold baths; uncovering.

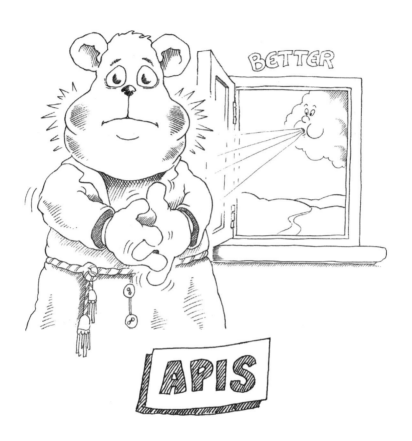

Argentum Nitricum
For symptoms arising from an over-active imagination. Great fear of heights.
Claustrophobia. Anticipatory states, easily panicked when a time is set, yet impulsive
and hurried. Headaches, often in one half of the head, from emotional causes and
overwork. Many stomach symptoms: painful distention and belching; diarrhoea after
eating and from apprehension.

Worse: Warmth and stuffiness; sweets and sugar; from emotions; left side.
Better: Cool fresh air; belching; from pressure (the headache).

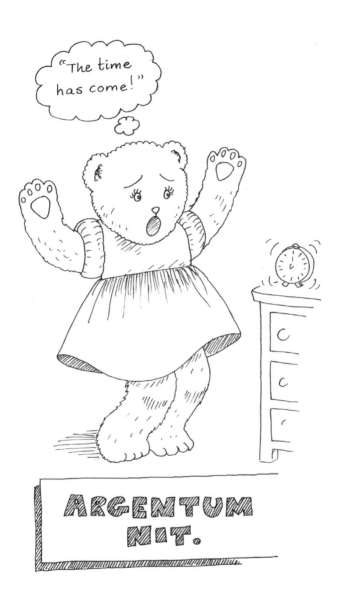

Arnica

Arnica is most useful for bruising, bleeding and shock caused by a fall or an accident. For operations, its pain-relief betters conventional drugs, and causes no drowsiness, constipation or other side-effects. In sports injuries, sprains and muscular strains, it is peerless. It can be given before extreme sports as a preventative, for instance before a marathon. Think of Arnica in cases where the patient starts from sleep in terror due to nightmares about a past accident or injury, or when they are too frightened to sleep because an old fear returns at night.

Persons needing Arnica say they are fine, even when they are not. It is a common experience to find an accident victim respond in this way, saying that they are perfectly well and in need of no assistance. Because their mind and body are in an over-sensitive state, they do not want to be touched and wish to be left alone. They may tell the doctor or carer to go away and that there is nothing wrong with them.

Physically, there is great soreness, and possibly a tendency to bleed. They may feel weak and exhausted, or they may be physically restless but mentally apathetic. They answer questions slowly, unwillingly or with great effort. If they are partly conscious, they answer correctly but then lapse back. The body and limbs ache as if bruised or beaten, and the bed feels too hard so that they have to change position often. Joints feel sprained.

Arnica has proven effective in treating people who bruise easily from the slightest knock.

Worse: Being touched; even the thought of being touched. For this reason they may tell you that they are well even when they are obviously traumatised.
Better: Lying down/head low; movement.

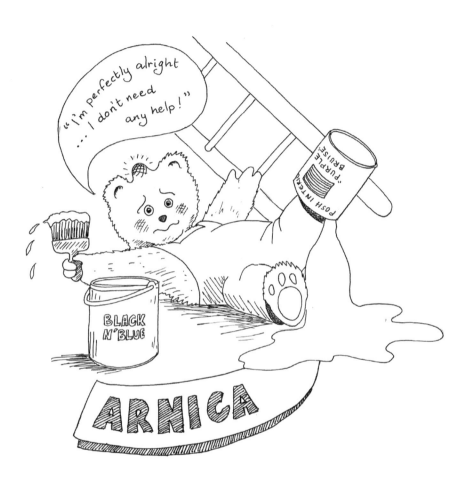

Arsenicum Album

May be needed for sudden collapse or when the weakness and exhaustion seems out of proportion to the complaint, as indeed is the person's concern over their health. Their life is full of anxiety: fearful they will lose what they have, unless they are extremely cautious. This makes them both restless and conscientious; cannot rest till things are in their proper place; anything that seems out of place troubles them. They are very cold, very worried and very hard to please; yet have a burning desire for someone to be around, for reassurance. This is because their worst, and usually unspoken, fear is that they will die alone. Their many fears and anxieties drive them to be restless, and if they wake at night, as they often do, usually between 2 and 3 a.m., then they may well get up and pace about. They complain of burning pains. They ask for water which they drink only in small sips. Should they catch a cold, then their runny noses will burn, or if they suffer diarrhoea, as from food poisoning, to which they are prone, it will be offensive and it will leave them feeling sore and totally exhausted.

Worse: After midnight; over-ripe fruit; bad meat/shellfish; becoming cold (but wants window open).
Better: Hot drinks; warmth; head propped up; sympathy and reassurance.

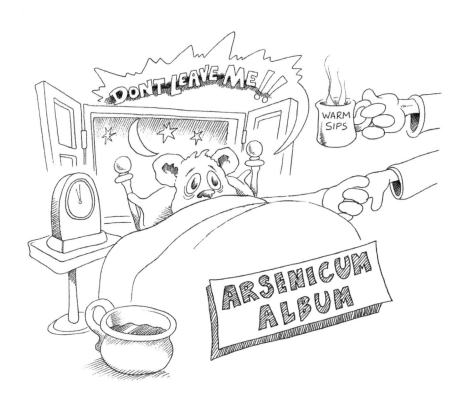

Belladonna

This person is red hot! Their heat radiates; with a high fever there is crimson redness. Often there is swelling and throbbing of affected or injured parts. Usually, the heat is concentrated in the head and torso and the feet and hands may be icy cold. The pupils may be dilated and a drugged expression may be evident, perhaps with hallucinations of wild animals or monsters. These fever terrors may be so intense that the child does not recognise the parent at whom it stares with dilated pupils in fright. They may even try to escape from you! The state can come on very suddenly and is often triggered by being out in the cold and wet, or after having a hair cut. Usually there is a marked lack of thirst or sweat.

Worse: 3 p.m. to midnight; sudden movement; light; touch; noise; lying down.
Better: Lying propped up; keeping still.

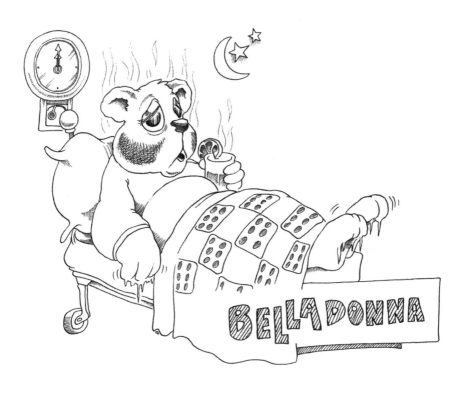

Bellis Perennis
This diminutive daisy of the field, common to the British Isles, shows characteristics of the British people that were particularly evident during the days of the Blitz: stoical; coming up smiling even while being repeatedly down-trodden.

Bellis is similar to Arnica in its action but has greatest affinity for injuries to deeper tissues, for instance after abdominal injury, surgery or miscarriage. It may be useful in cases of bruising where bumps remain after a bruise has cleared or where Arnica has cleared the bruising but a lump persists. Bellis is also useful when the body has been overworked and stretched beyond its capacity. Strained muscles or tendons from weight lifting or in endurance athletes such as marathon runners come into this category, as do the stiff and sore bodies of gardeners. Bellis is also one of the remedies that can be very useful for falls on the tailbone, when you might also consider Hypericum.

These people remain cheerful despite pains and/or feeling unwell, or conversely may be irritable, weepy and desire solitude. Pushing helpers away is a key-note symptom of Arnica which applies to Bellis too.

WORSE: If hot, for cold drinks, cold wind and becoming wet with cold water. Touch. Warm bed. Injuries and sprains.
BETTER: Continued motion. Open air. After eating

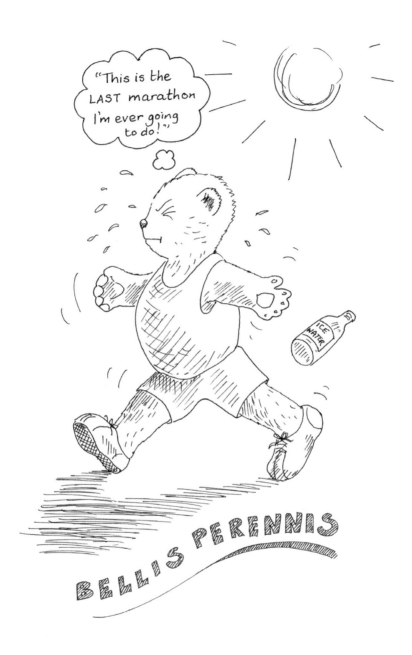

Bryonia

This is a bear with a sore head, whose headaches are so terrible that any movement, even of the eyes, is unbearable. Movement aggravates is a general theme of this remedy. When they have any pain, which is described as bursting or stitching, they will often feel better for holding on to it, to prevent movement. They have a marked desire to be left alone and are very irritable. They drink copious amounts of cold water (and want you around to provide these) but their lips and tongue will still feel dry. The mental symptom, which is often at the root of their acute symptoms, is money worries and an irrational fear of being destitute. This really can play on their minds and might force them out of bed to work despite their obvious suffering.

Worse: Least movement; eating; hot weather; morning on waking; 9 p.m.
Better: Lying on painful part; rest.

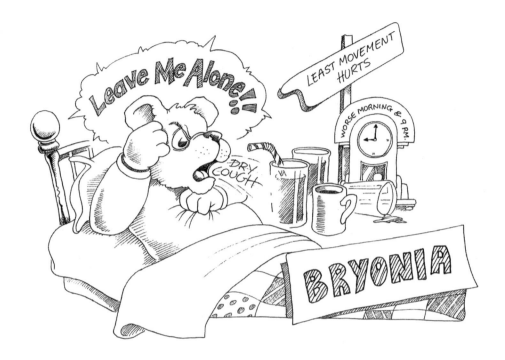

Calcarea Carbonica

If your child is a late developer, has been slow to teeth, crawl and walk, a plodder not a pusher, then this could be their constitutional remedy. They are usually plump and easy going, happy to watch others, or to play by themselves. Their heads may sweat at night, and their bowel movements and perspiration usually smells sour. They can also go without passing a motion for several days, without any apparent ill effects. They like bland foods, especially soft boiled eggs, milk and ice cream, although these may disagree with them. They generally dislike meat. They like cold food and though they are chilly, they do not enjoy hot baths. Cold weather can aggravate them, and they like their hats and scarves. They are prone to coughs and colds, swollen glands, tonsillitis and ear infections.

Although they may be slow learners, these children are determined and independent and can be very stubborn. They may suffer from nerves and fear when they are unwell. They are afraid of the dark, and may wake up screaming from nightmares; also they have fear of some animals, for example mice and dogs. They avoid the rough and tumble of the playground; at sport, they are apt to sprain their ankles. They are not outspoken in class, fearing that others will notice their confusion. Older children may develop a fear of death and become fascinated by religious ideas and the supernatural. This remedy should be considered if the child has had repeated fevers that have been helped by Belladonna.

Worse: Mental and physical effort; cold/wet weather; on waking; morning and after midnight; full and new moon.
Better: Lying down; dry weather; hot applications; rubbing.

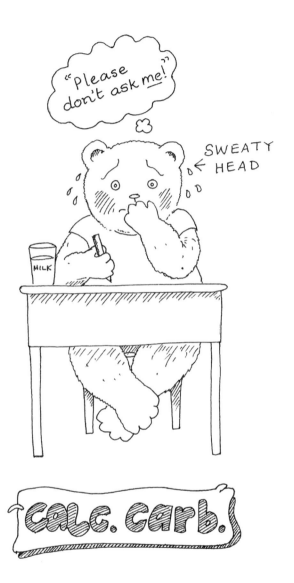

Calendula

Calendula is available as a cream as well as in the potentised form and we recommend you have both. It is the most remarkable healing agent where the pain is excessive and out of all proportion to the injury. Useful for open wounds, grazes, and parts that will not heal, scalp wounds, ulcers, etc. Promotes healthy and rapid healing. Ensure the affected part is completely clean before applying the cream, or use the infusion for this purpose.

Calendula is great on all types of wounds and helps stop bleeding it may also prevent the development of disfiguring scars from torn and jagged wounds. In addition, the infusion of the remedy may soothe eczema. Calendula is prescribed internally and externally for leg and varicose ulcers, post-operative wounds, and ruptured muscles or tendons. Calendula may be used to treat torn perineal tissues following childbirth, joint wounds where there is loss of synovial fluid, and bleeding in the gums after a tooth extraction.

From Dorothy Shepherd: "It is the best herbal wound dressing and antiseptic that I know. Alack and alas! that so few, even keen homoeopaths, appreciate its value as such. I worked for years in various homoeopathic hospitals and never saw it used; we used the same lotions, tinctures and dressings as the orthodox hospitals. Calendula is wonderful for wounds with or without loss of substance, with sharp cutting pains, redness, rawness, and sometimes stinging pains during febrile heat - then it acts like magic and promotes rapid healing."

Worse: In damp, heavy, cloudy weather.
Better: Resting, peace, gentle exercise.

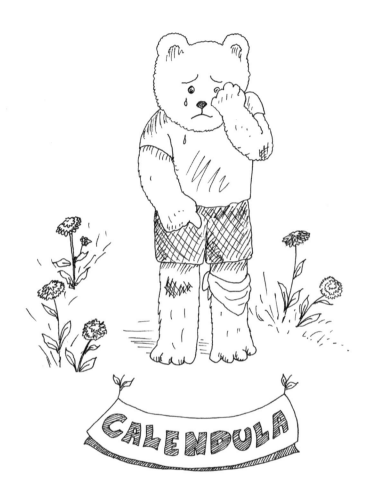

Cantharis

This is the first remedy to think of after a scald or burn, where the affected area is red and blistered; so painful that it drives the person to distraction. This remedy is also good for sunburn and for insect bites where the pain is intensely burning. The pains may also be cutting, raw and smarting and can be due to acute inflammations, not only on the skin, but in the urinary and sexual organs too, for instance after forced sex (cf. Staphisagria). Violent burning and cutting pains in bladder and urethra and constant, intolerable urging; before, during and after urination. Pain in the bladder is worse drinking even the smallest sip of water, or from drinking coffee.

Worse: Urinating; drinking cold drinks; bright objects; sound of water; touch on voice box; coffee.
Better: Warmth; rest; rubbing.

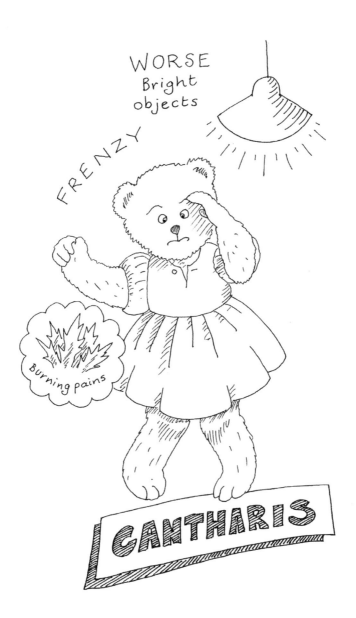

Carbo Vegetabilis

The medical use of charcoal (Carbo Vegetabilis) in treating abdominal wind is well known. The flatulence is extreme with a feeling of great fullness. They cannot bear tight clothing around their waist and they are temporarily better by bringing up wind. Other keynote symptoms of this remedy are extreme weakness, low vitality, sluggishness, indolence, coldness; sensation as if the blood had stagnated; blueness from lack of oxygen, better for fanning and desire for fresh air with icy coldness of limbs. Causes may be shock, a heart attack or accident or the after effects of exhausting diseases including a protracted bout of whooping cough. This remedy has been dubbed, 'the corpse reviver'.

Worse: Warm wet weather (sultry weather); depletions; high living and rich food; extremes of weather; old age; suppressions.
Better: Burping; cool air; being fanned; putting feet up.

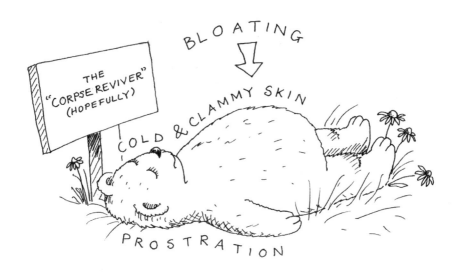

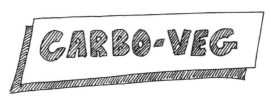

Caulophyllum

Squaw root or Blue Cohosh is a remedy from North America used by native American women to ease the pains of menstruation and childbirth. It was also used to help establish or strengthen uterine contractions and bring about a smooth delivery.

Caulophyllum has a well established reputation for toning up the uterus and hastening the delivery of babies that are overdue. It is a powerful agent for the prevention of premature labour and miscarriage too, providing the pains are of a spasmodic nature. Useful for painful, ineffective contractions i.e. when the cervix is not dilating, and also if labour stops altogether. Also useful after the birth if the uterus does not contract properly, or if the placenta is not fully expelled, or if after-pains are unbearably painful, extending across the lower abdomen to the groins.

Also useful if a woman, before or during menses, experiences a mix of the following: chilliness, vertigo, nausea, lower back pain. Pains are drawing, cramping, shooting and erratic. Symptoms are typically accompanied by thirst, chilliness, exhaustion and trembling.

The person may be irritable, nervous or excitable.

WORSE: Open air. Pregnancy. Suppressed menses. Motion. Evening. Coffee.
BETTER: Warmth.

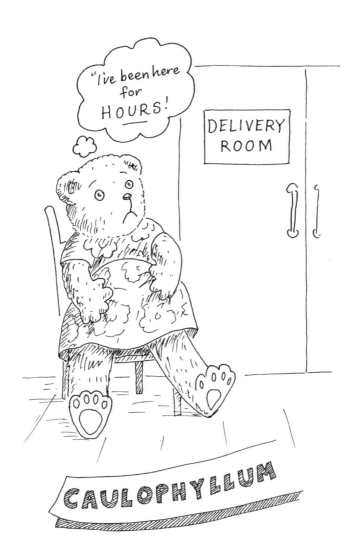

Causticum

At the emotional level these people cannot tolerate any injustice and are susceptible to intense and long held grief that metaphorically burns into them. At the physical level burning pains are characteristic, as if raw, sore or open. Indeed, Causticum is a major player in the treatment of second and third degree burns. To continue the parallels: these people have difficulties with authority because they identify with the holocausted outcasts, the victims in society, and they tend to be idealistic or revolutionary: they can literally burn with fanaticism. If they are unable to realise their ideals, then they may develop diseases characterised by tightening, hardening, 'holding on', followed by weakness and gradual paralysis that can play out emotionally, mentally and physically.

Emotionally: they suffer and weep easily from sympathy with others. Their ailments can often be traced back to numerous griefs. They tend to internalised like Natrum Mur. They suffer from the injustices in society, and may become fighters for a cause, whistle blowers, selflessly working to help the poor and the oppressed.
Mentally: they can develop fears that something terrible will happen. They are anxious for others, always on tenterhooks, always checking where a loved one has gone, when they will return. They may suffer weakness of memory, a characteristic feeling they had forgotten something. Forebodings, worse twilight and at night.
Physically: there may be twitching or facial paralysis (mainly right-sided), paralysis of the bladder, paralysis of vocal cords, drooping of upper eye-lids. Stammering on account of excitement or anger. Burning pains, like raw flesh, as from an open wound. Sensation as if muscles and tendons were too short. Involuntary urination when sneezing, coughing, walking, blowing the nose, during first sleep, from becoming cold. Dry, deep cough, can't cough deep enough to raise mucus. Symptoms tend to develop gradually.

Worse: Cold; raw winds; drafts. Extremes of temperature. Stooping. Suppressions. Coffee. 3-4 am or evening. Exertion. Clear weather. Motion of carriage. While perspiring. New moon. Getting wet. Entering a warm room from the open air.
Better: Sips of cold drinks. Washing. Warmth of bed. Gentle motion. Warm air. Damp, wet weather. Craves smoked things, smoked meat.

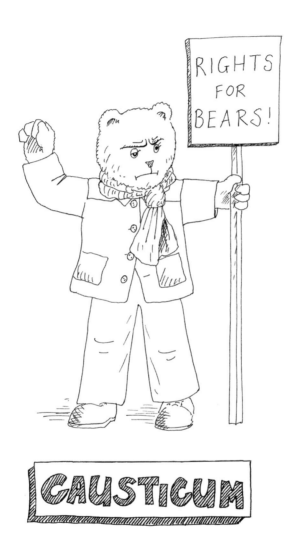

CAUSTICUM

Chamomilla
This is the most commonly indicated teething remedy. One cheek red and hot, other cheek pale and cold. The child screams constantly and wants to be carried everywhere.

The pain is unbearable. They will demand various things, and then throw them away; they are impossible to please. They do not even want you to look at them. Diarrhoea may have the appearance of chopped egg and spinach. But this is equally a brilliant pain reliever for adults when the key idea, 'cannot bear it' is there, such as in toothache, when irritability and rudeness predominate. Ailments arising from anger, coffee and narcotics.

Worse: Teething; Cold air; being looked at.
Better: Being carried; cold compress.

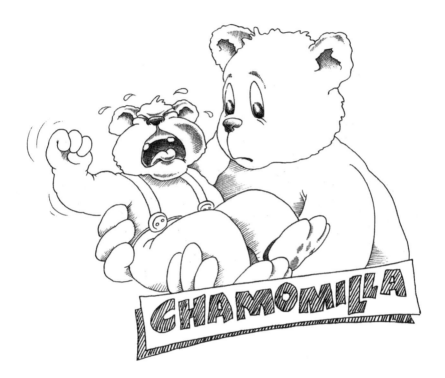

Chelidonium

This is a wasteland plant, related to the wild poppy, and like it has a latex that runs freely when the plant is injured. Unlike the poppy its latex is bright yellow-orange and is bitter and burning. In therapeutics it is best known for gall-stones, with pain under the right shoulder-blade.

Chelidonium is an important liver remedy useful in conditions like hepatitis, malaria and liver damage from alcohol abuse. It is also useful for gastric and intestinal catarrhs, a loose, rattling cough and right-sided pneumonia. The skin is likely to be sallow or jaundiced and may be itchy.

There may be dizziness, nausea and vomiting. Pains are felt in the liver area, often extending to the back and shoulders, or in the stomach. The pains are aching, sharp, shooting or stitching, and tend to be on the right side.

The person will usually be dull, lethargic and gloomy. They may feel restless or anxious and be averse to talking or any mental exertion. You may get the feeling that they have suffered intensely and cope by shutting off into dullness. They are generally practical, strong-minded and down to earth people who can be domineering.

WORSE: 4am or 4pm. Motion. Cough. Touch. Changes of weather. Windy weather. Heat or hot applications. Warm room. Lying on right side. Early morning. Cold food and cold drinks.
BETTER: Hot food. Eating dinner. Hot milk, coffee or other hot drinks. Pressure. Hot bath. Bending backward.

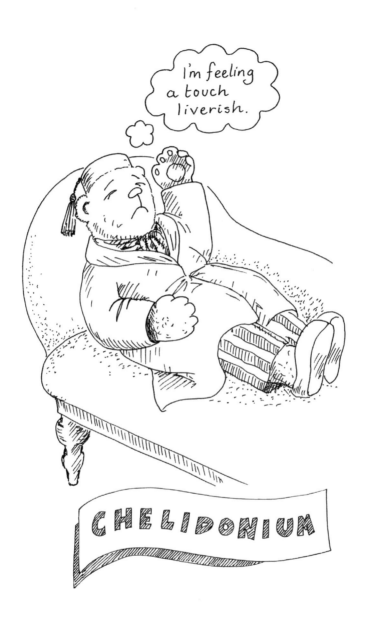

Cimicifuga

Squaw root; Black Cohosh. Another remedy from North America used by native American women in childbirth. During labour: shivering in the first stage; convulsions from nervous excitement; cervix rigid; pains severe and spasmodic, aggravated by least noise. Helps dilate the cervix in labour.

A useful remedy for nerve and muscle pain, neuritis and muscle hypersensitivity. Also for ovarian and uterine ailments, especially dysmenorrhea. Pains are cramping, squeezing and twisting. Symptoms move around a great deal and there is much soreness or a bruised feeling. The left side is more often affected.There may be great weakness or stiffness in the limbs. Muscular rheumatism; stiff neck, drawing head back; can't turn the head. Headache pressing outward or upward, as if top of head would fly off, or into eyes or down nape into spine.

The person may look very pale and feel cold to the touch. They may be extremely restless and loquacious. They may sigh a great deal and feel miserable or fearful. Sensation, as if a heavy, black cloud had settled all over her and enveloped her head, so that all is darkness and confusion. There may be a fear of insanity. Fear during pregnancy.

WORSE: During menses. During labour. Emotions. Alcohol. Damp, cold weather. Wind. Drafts. Change of weather. Sitting. Taking cold. Motion. Excitement. Menopause.
BETTER: Warm wraps. Open air. Pressure. Gentle, continued motion. Eating. Grasping thighs. Rest.

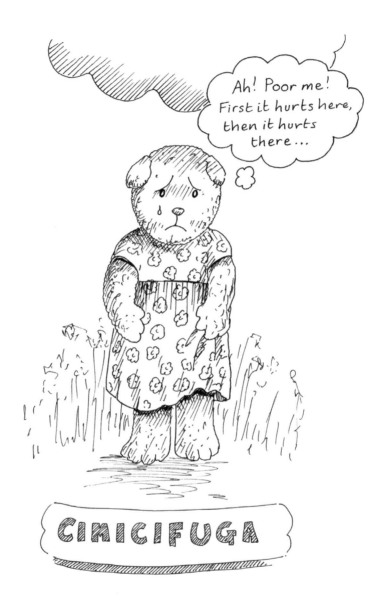

Chinchona Officinalis
This is the very first remedy ever proved by Hahnemann. He was living in Edinburgh earning money by translating at Edinburgh University when he decided to try China for himself to see what happens – the rest, as they say, is history. Like Carbo Veg. this remedy is useful for excessive bloating of the belly where bringing up wind does not bring relief. Often the troubles, of whatever nature, come on after loss of fluids, this could be from blood loss, excessive menstruation, prolonged breastfeeding or extreme diarrhoea, which cause exhaustion, weakness, headaches with bursting, throbbing pain, extending from the back to the whole head; stomach disturbances; anaemia. People needing China are worse for light touch, rubbing or caressing, but better for hard pressure. They suffer from general oversensitivity, perhaps even from paranoia, feeling themselves to be harassed, unfortunate, thinking that the world is hostile. They may be sleepless from over abundant ideas and plans.

Worse: Loss of fluids; touch; regularly returning symptoms; alternate days; wind; cold; summer and autumn.
Better: Hard pressure; loose clothing; bending double; warmth.

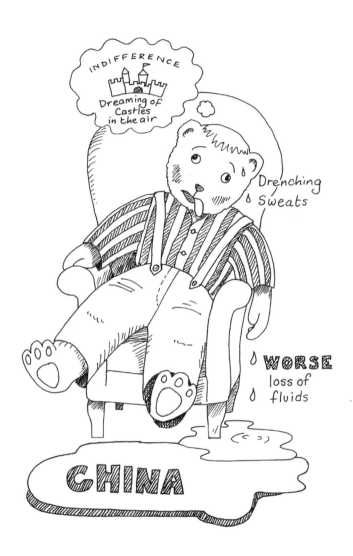

Cocculus

A very useful remedy for travel sickness. Characteristically there is vertigo and dizziness with nausea and vomiting. There may also be headaches and muscle weakness. It may be useful in early pregnancy nausea/morning sickness, especially if the person cannot bear the sight or thought of food. There may also be a one-sided paralysis, with numbness in the limbs. It is a useful remedy for sleep problems where there is frequent waking.

The person may have a sensation of hollowness or emptiness in the abdomen and will not want to eat, but there may be a desire for cold drinks. The person is very sensitive to noise and odours. They may feel angry, on edge, but will typically make out that everything is okay. They tend to suppress negativity and anger (like Staphisagria).

Sympathetic to others; anxious for the welfare of others. Cocculus is useful in cases where night watching over children, or sick or elderly has undermined strength – this is a key-note of the remedy.

WORSE: Loss of sleep. Talking. Laughing. Crying. Emotions. Motion. Coffee. After drinking. Cold. Open air. Eating. Thought and smell of food. Menses. Pregnancy. Smoking. Exertion. Touch.
BETTER: Warmth. Lying quietly.

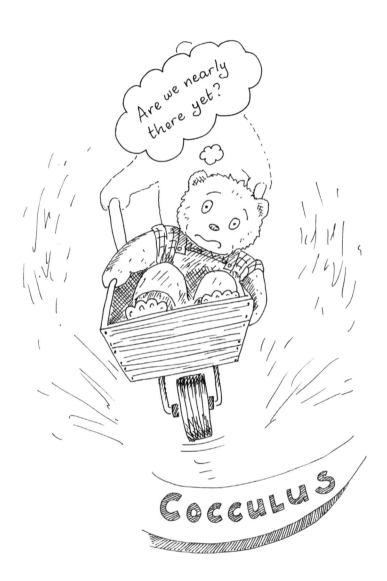

Drosera

One of a trio of remedies that have a strong effect on croup. Hepar Sulph. and Spongia are the other two. Drosera is indicated for croup, whooping cough and other lung disorders that produce these symptoms: a maddening tickling in the throat with spasmodic coughing that can lead to vomiting, the person struggles to breathe, and has cold sweats. Stitching pains in the chest worse for coughing. The coughing spasms come every 2 to 3 hours. The patient can be frightened of being alone when ill, yet may be irrationally suspicious that friends and family are deceiving them at the same time.

Worse: After midnight; lying down; warmth; cold food; laughing; vomiting.
Better: Open air.

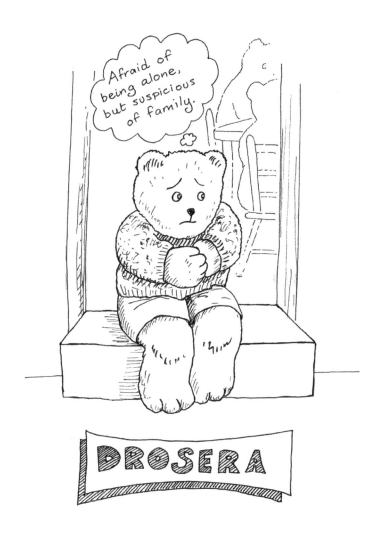

Eupatorium

This person will complain of aching all over, and may feel as if their bones are broken, particularly in their neck, back and legs. The ache extends even to their eyeballs. They have shaking chills but desire ice cream, and acid drinks; beware of cold water though - it makes them vomit.

Worse: Cold air; 7 to 9 a.m.; movement; smell or sight of food.
Better: After vomiting; conversation.

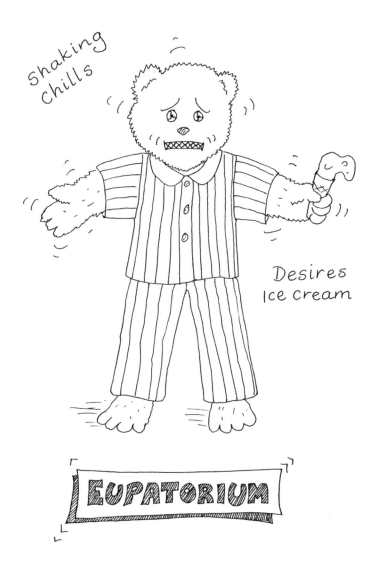

Shaking Chills

Desires Ice cream

EUPATORIUM

Euphrasia
Common name is Eyebright. A useful remedy for acute conjunctivitis, as well as for hay fever, catarrhal colds, headaches (temple area), measles, influenza and coughs.

With eye symptoms there may be photophobia and smarting or burning pains, itchiness, redness, sticky eyes and yellow discharge (conjunctivitis). Whereas there is an acrid discharge from the eyes there may be an equally copious but bland discharge from the nose. The membranes inside the nostrils are swollen and there is much sneezing and breathlessness.

The person may be feeling anxious, confused, angry and definitely will not want to make idle conversation.

WORSE: Sunlight, wind, warmth, evening, indoors, morning on rising, in bed, moisture, touch, wind.
BETTER: Open air, winking, wiping eyes, darkness, lying down.

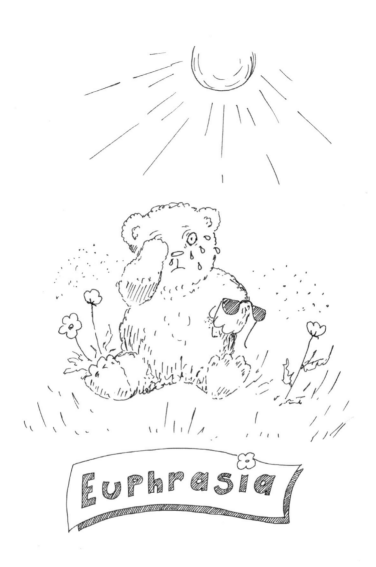

Ferrum Phos.
For the early stages of many illnesses which may take several days to develop. They tend to be flopped out. The person is flushed, but not feverish. Face alternately red and pale. They are irritable, excitable, but changeable, and may become depressed. This person will usually have been very affectionate, yet strong willed, even dictatorial, when healthy.

Worse: 4 to 6 a.m.; during the night; motion; noise; cold drinks.
Better: Slow movement; lying down.

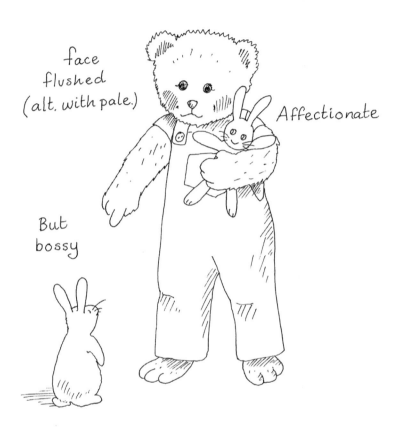

face
flushed
(alt. with pale.)

Affectionate

But
bossy

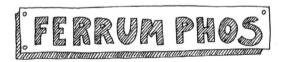

FERRUM PHOS

Gelsemium

May be indicated when the patient has been on the receiving end of some bad or unexpected news, or has anxiety over a forthcoming event or ordeal, such as an exam or court appearance. They feel they may not be able to cope. Their symptoms are diarrhoea, loss of appetite, thirstlessness and they do not want to move or talk. Even opening their eyes is too much effort. The onset of these symptoms is quite slow. It is a commonly indicated flu remedy with shivers up and down the spine, a great sense of heaviness and fatigue, a burning discharge from the nose and a tickling cough which is better near a fire or heater.

Worse: Emotion and anticipation; thinking; damp weather; sun; lying propped up.
Better: Keeping quiet; open air; urinating; sweating.

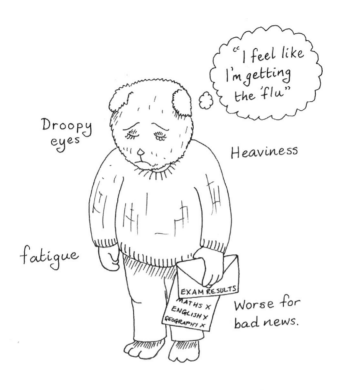

Hepar Sulph.

This remedy is useful to know for many ailments, including croup, coughs, wheezing. Hepar Sulph. has been known to cure asthma after eczema has been suppressed by creams, such as those containing hydrocortisone. This is because it stimulates the body to reverse such suppression and to bring the now internalised trouble to the surface. It also has the capacity to ripen an abscess or a boil, to bring it to a head from which it may discharge and then heal. Hepar Sulph. helps constitutions which are prone to festering; even the slightest injury suppurates. Recurrent attacks of suppurating tonsillitis; of chronic middle ear infections. The pains are stitching and stabbing; splinter-like. The sweat and discharges are sour or smell like old cheese. These people have a strong craving for acids (vinegar, pickles) and pungent flavours. Their complaints may appear after they have been out in a cold, dry wind. Their skin is very sensitive to touch, and they are generally extremely sensitive to drafts.

In general they are hypersensitive customers, as if they had weak barriers; they easily feel worried that hostile outside influences will affect them. Even during hot weather, they will feel the cold intensely and extending a limb from the bedclothes will be enough to set off a coughing fit. They are acutely sensitive to emotional stresses. Horrible stories affect them as if they had suffered such things themselves. When ill they are hurried and irritable like a volcano about to blow. People needing this remedy easily feel offended, for instance contradiction gives rise to feelings of injury and then they over react. They can be violent (especially from pain which is often stabbing in character), and then they may have sudden impulses to stab and kill.

Worse: Dry cold air/slight draft, least uncovering; touch; lying on painful side; night; noise; exertion.
Better: Warmth; warm/damp weather; wrapping up.

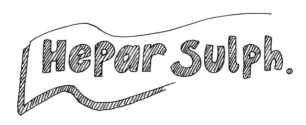

Hepar Sulph.

(Worse for the least draught.)

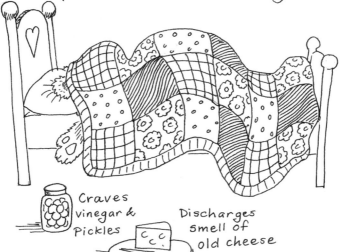

Craves vinegar & Pickles

Discharges smell of old cheese

Hypericum

One of the main remedies for injuries to nerves, especially of fingers, toes, coccyx and nail beds. Crushed fingers, especially tips. Excessive painfulness is a guiding symptom to its use. Punctured and lacerated wounds. Prevents lockjaw. Relieves pain after operations. Spasms after every injury. Injured nerves from animal bites. Tetanus. Neuritis, tingling, burning and numbness.

Worse: Injury; penetrating wounds; concussion; shock; bruises; forceps delivery; touch; exertion; cold air; change of weather; foggy weather; motion.
Better: Bending back; lying on stomach; rubbing.

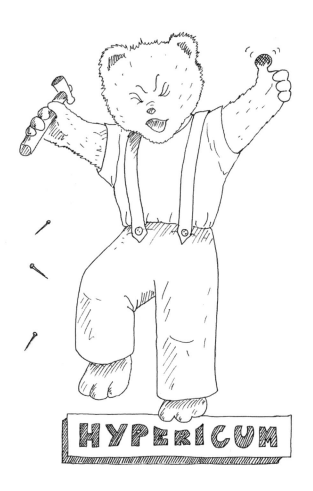

Ignatia

This is the first remedy to think of for teenagers, or anyone becoming hysterical after bad news, grief, fright, worry, disappointed love, jealousy. It is as though this person had put all their eggs into one basket, so that if the basket should fall, an 'end of the world' crisis must ensue. Affects the nervous system producing on the physical level spasms, twitches and tremors, and contradictory symptoms such as sensation of a lump in the throat better for swallowing. On the mental and emotional level this is seen in hysteria with emotional outbursts that are very quickly controlled: only tears in eyes but no sobbing, or just short sobs, or incessant sighing, constant swallowing, twitching around the mouth, silent brooding. They may go off food or eat incessantly.

Worse: Emotions; grief; worry; fright; shock; loss of loved one; air; odours; coffee; tobacco; yawning; waking; standing.
Better: Movement; urinating; company; swallowing; deep breathing; eating.

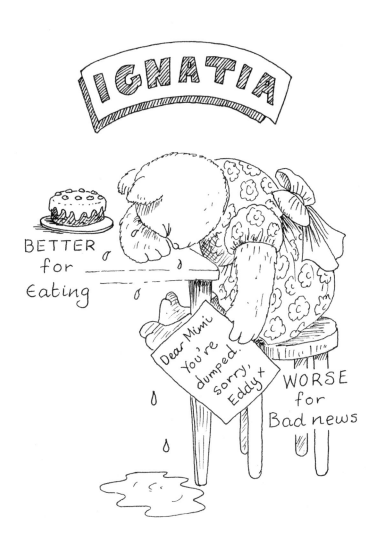

Ipecacuanha

This remedy is used in large doses in conventional medicine as an emetic (to induce vomiting), but in homeopathic potency to cure persistent nausea. Ask if this person has overeaten rich foods, particularly pork or ice cream? Perhaps they have been in the sun, or been made angry or indignant over a situation (that makes them feel like vomiting). Are they complaining of feeling constantly nauseous or being constantly sick, or do they have an excruciating stomach ache, and are sulking, irritable and easily offended? If they have these symptoms together with no appetite or thirst, a noticeable improvement from open air, and worsening when in a stuffy room, and a clean tongue - think Ipecacuanha.

Worse: Slightest movement; overeating; nausea worse from stooping.
Better: Open air; rest; cold drinks.

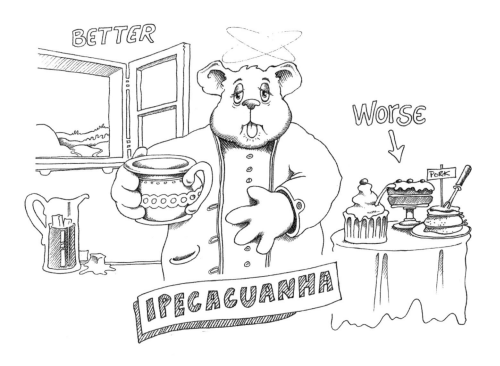

Kali Carbonicum
This remedy often comes up during childbirth when the following symptoms are present: inefficient labour pains which begin in the back and pass off down the buttocks rather than spreading round the sides; 'back labours' with a nagging lower backache between and during contractions; sharp cutting pains across the lower back; lower back pain that is better for firm pressure or rubbing The whole body feels heavy and broken down, and any exertion requires great effort. Pains are stitching, throbbing or darting.

The abdomen may be bloated with wind. Exhaustion. Restlessness and thirst. She feels the pulsation of all the arteries, even down to the toes. Feeling of emptiness in the whole body, as if it were hollow. Perspires easily on slight exertion. A useful remedy for congestion and cold symptoms, including congestive headaches, nasal colds, sore throats, chesty coughs. Chilly when out of doors from the least cool air. Extreme sensitivity to drafts. Nose obstructed in room; clear in open air, but returns on re-entering room.

Particularly suitable if the person is anaemic or has lost a great deal of fluid and/ or vitality following illness (like China), or for those who often catch a cold. When afflicted they typically suffer very fluent discharge with frequent sneezing. They often have watery swellings under the eyes. With throat conditions there is difficulty swallowing and a severe sticking pain (like Hepar sulph). Choking hoarseness and loss of voice from a lump sensation in the throat. Tormenting, dry cough; gets nothing up. Wakes at 2 or 3 am with great dryness of throat, or asthmatic breathing, coughs for an hour, with gagging and scanty expectoration.

This person may be irritable and quarrelsome yet is very prone to anxiety and wants company. When in health they are conscientious, have a strong sense of duty and like to ensure everything and everybody is safely under their watchful control.

WORSE: Cold, drafts, touch, noise, night, early morning, being alone, loss of fluids, lying on affected side
BETTER: Warmth, open air, eructations, soup, firm pressure.

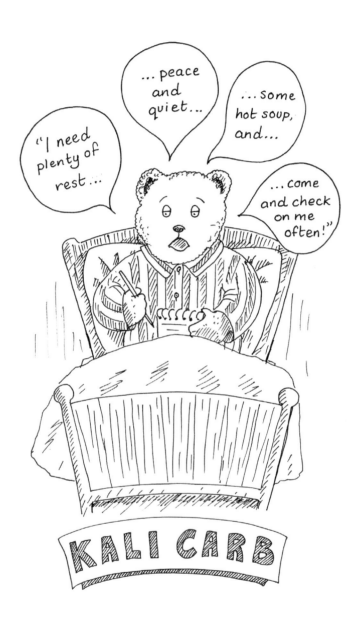

Kali Phosphoricum

Kali phos is often recommended for exhaustion and weak contractions during labour, especially if there are no other distinguishing symptoms. Elsewhere the history is often one of grief, mental shock, overwork, a debilitating illness, or caring for others for too long. The senses become dull and she cannot use her mind anymore; she is worn out, slow to answer questions and apathetic. She may desire solitude.

Crushing headache. Headache from top of head to right eye. Menstrual headache, before and during the flow. Hair loss. Sensation of sticks in the eyes; of sand in eyes; as if eyes were dry. Rumbling in bowels; flatulence. Painless, non-debililtating diarrhea. Urine very yellow. Stitching all through the pelvis and uterus. Bloody discharge during pregnancy. Night pains during pregnancy. Palpitation. Better from belching. Desires fruity, juicy and refreshing things. Loss of appetite from grief. Chilly. Very tired feeling.

WORSE: Emotions, grief, mental shock, bad news, worry, too much study, loss of fluids, cold air, becoming cold, cold drinks, physical exertion, talking, standing, ascending stairs, milk, winter, uncovering head, noise, being alone.
BETTER: Warmth, gentle motion, stool, short sleep.

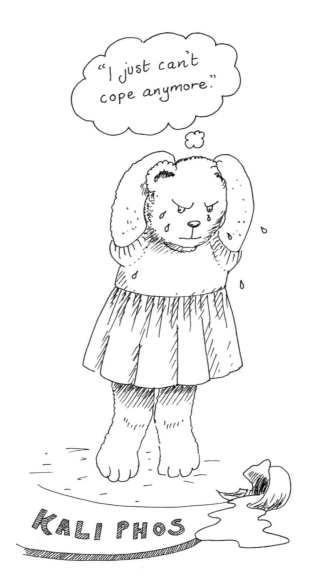

Lachesis

These people are intense. They are also loquacious. There is so much going on inside that needs to be expressed, they just cannot keep it in. Often they are so talkative that it is impossible for anyone to get a word in edgewise. If the outlet for these intense emotions has been suppressed, then the outward presentation may be soft, pleasant and introverted. When this happens, there are feelings of inferiority with hidden envy and a frustrated, critical tendency toward almost everyone around them. In either of these presentations they unerringly sense the vulnerable spots of others and may strike at them. The extrovert types are endowed with a sarcastic wit and can be mercilessly cutting. Teenagers have high sexual energy. They can become controlling of their partner and, if carried too far, this may develop into obsessive possessiveness.

The Lachesis child is usually unable to effectively control their strong emotions. This child may become jealous of a new sibling and will openly declare that he hates a younger brother or sister. They may also be possessive of friends and demand that they are paid particular attention. This child seems to have a precocious awareness of the people around them and instinctively uses this to gain the upper hand. They cannot bear to be under the authority of another person and do not tolerate restrictions. Physical pathologies develop when they cannot gain the upper hand.

These people are warm blooded physically as well as emotionally. They are also worse for external warmth. They have many circulatory disturbances, palpitations and violent hot flushes. They can develop purple, bluish discolorations. Their ailments tend to be left-sided or after beginning on the left extend to the right. Choking from clothing around neck, from slight pressure or touch. They are worse during and after a long sleep and worse in the morning on waking. Paroxysms of sneezing in hay fever, especially worse after sleeping. Left-sided quinsy, extending to the right side, worse warm drinks, better cold drinks.

Worse: After sleep; they sleep into aggravation; morning; becoming heated; spring and autumn; summer sun; extremes of temperature; empty swallowing. Worse for pressure of touch or clothing; noise; start and close of menses; 'never well since menopause.'; suppressed discharges; alcohol.
Better: Open air; free secretions; hard pressure; bathing the affected part; cold drinks; discharges especially menses (as soon as the flow starts); worse before menses.

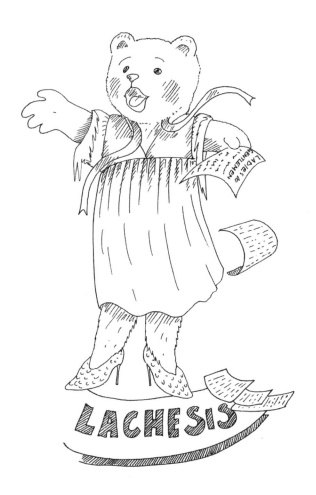

LACHESIS

Ledum

A good remedy for puncture wounds and black eyes. Shown to have anti-tetanus properties. Useful for treating deep penetrating wounds such as those caused by nails, and bites from both animals and insects. Tick bites and consequent Lymes disease have been helped with Ledum.

If tetanus threatens after wounds think first of Hypericum, especially after torn nails, or lacerated parts rich in nerves; when accompanied with the sensation of bruising think of Arnica; when open lacerations and cuts, think of Calendula.

For Ledum, the injured area will become swollen, mottled and blue and feel cold to the touch, however the person feels that it is hot. Relief comes from cold applications. Pains are sticking, tearing and throbbing. There may be feelings of nausea, intoxication or vertigo.

The person may be averse to company and feel hateful and resentful.

WORSE: Heat, motion, night, alcohol, eggs, walking, lying down (cough).
BETTER: Cold applications, rest, eating (headache).

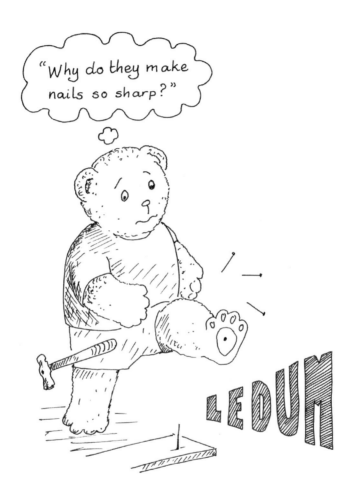

Lycopodium Clavatum

Do your child's coughs develop easily into bronchitis? Are they cross in the mornings, and have a large head and a thin, weak body? Do they need regular meals, or feel faint, and do they prefer hot food and drinks and love sweets? Do they tend to fill up easily and can suffer from wind, bloatedness and constipation? They are chilly, yet love fresh air and will not keep a hat on? Do their swollen glands and tonsillitis tend to be more prominent on the right side? Do they get crabby at 4 in the afternoon? Lycopodium children also prefer books to football boots, and are happy to be alone, reading, as long as they know someone else is around. They have fears of the dark, of being alone, and of facing new situations, meeting new people, and will try and avoid this challenge. As a result of this timidity, and also because of the physical weakness, Lycopodium children may be averse to play, shunning sports and games. The Lycopodium teenager however, being too arrogant to admit to his lack of self-confidence in facing new situations and meeting new people, will try and compensate for his inner weakness by surrounding himself with people whom he can dominate. He creates around him a world in which others accept his authority. His dictatorial attitude is however, confined to within the safety of his domain, and when he steps outside he is still timid. And so he seldom ventures out, rather he seeks only to expand his safe domain further, bringing more and more people under his control.

Worse: Right side; 4 to 8 p.m; morning; after midnight; cold and cold food or drinks.
Better: Cool open air; uncovering; especially the head; warm drinks; wet weather.

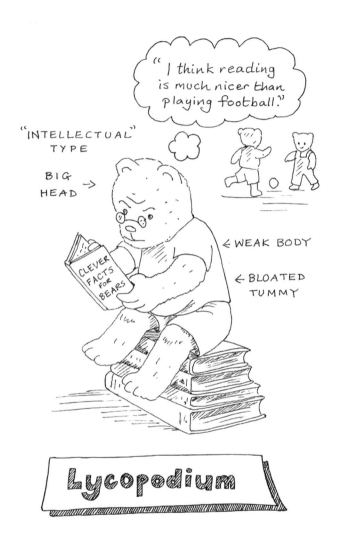

Magnesia Phosphorica

The characteristic pains are sharp, neuralgic, cramping, cutting, piercing, knife-like, shooting; lightning-like in coming and going; rapidly changing place. Great dread of cold air; of uncovering; of touching affected parts. There is general improvement of all pains by the application of local heat. Whether toothache, menstrual cramps or sciatic pain, a hot-water bottle and rest will help.

Laments all the time about the pains; sobbing, crying. Sensation as of a strong shock of electricity passing from head to all parts of the body. Spasms or twitching. Menstrual colic. Severe dysmenorrhoea. Tires very easily, even from talking.

The person may be sensitive or nervous and not want to talk about their pain, alternatively may talk constantly about their pains! They are likely to be restless and anxious. The pain exhausts them and their sleep may be disturbed because of it.

WORSE: Cold, uncovering, touch, night, motion.
BETTER: Heat, firm pressure, doubling up.

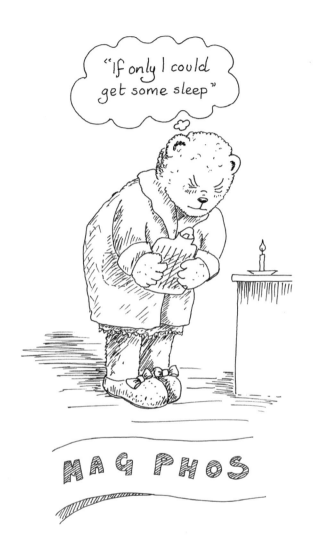

Mercurius

Just about everything aggravates this person: heat, cold, night, covering up, uncovering and so on. Their temperature is unstable and so are their moods. At their worst, they feel so angry they could kill. They can have a keen sense of personal injustice, feeling that the world is their enemy and out to get them. They can develop an 'I'll get them before they get me' attitude, or they can feel defeated and depleted. They have a bad taste in their mouths and offensive breath, even the discharge from their nose smells, and their saliva stains the pillow yellow. They are very thirsty and sweaty and dribble a lot at night.

Worse: Heat; cold; damp; extremes of temperature; warmth of bed; uncovering; night.
Better: Rest; lying down.

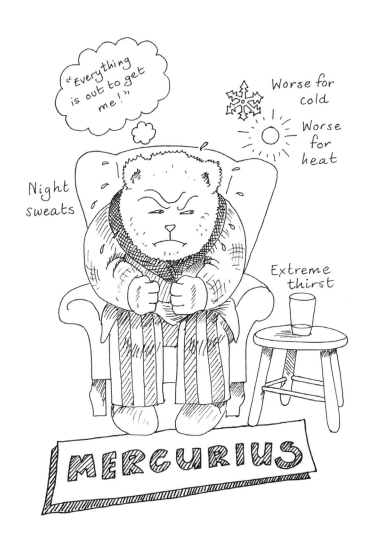

Natrum Muriaticum
These children often suffer from headaches, particularly during the school day. Another of their common symptoms is colds, with a clear mucus discharge, a little like the white of an egg, with much sneezing. They are sensitive to emotional atmospheres and also to their physical environment, and may develop allergies, especially hay fever, and can have cracked lips and frequent cold sores. Often they have a craving for salt, which they liberally add to their meals, and aversion to bread. They are sensitive to the sun, as exposure tends to bring on a headache (worse 10 a.m.).

Sensitivity runs through their homeopathic picture: they are very easily hurt, and because they are aware of their own vulnerability they are careful not to hurt another's feelings. Teenagers crave a romantic, loving relationship and because of their vulnerability they are led into a situation in which they easily feel that their trust or faith has been betrayed. Hence they become reserved and unapproachable. She believes that there is something wrong with her: either she is not good looking enough or she has not done enough, and this is why the other person will be disappointed and leave her. This makes her do her best to be nurturing and caring, makes her go out of her way for others. But when hurt, she withdraws completely with aversion to consolation. There is bitterness. She dwells on past disagreeable occurrences. She plays sad songs in the privacy of her room.

Nat. Mur. people would find it easier to write a letter or a poem to a friend who had hurt them, than speak to them directly, but they would probably not post it. This alternates with a desire for a physical relationship. Thus we find contradictory symptoms in these people. In order to avoid a love disappointment they may enter into a relationship where, from the beginning, there is no expectation of total commitment, like falling in love with a married man; silent, one-sided love. This is a major love disappointment and grief remedy and needs to be compared with its more acute sister remedy, Ignatia. With regard to fears, they are often claustrophobic (shut into their own psychic space), and can develop an obsession about robbers. Strangers breaking in finds its corollary in the key symptom, worse for consolation, for these people are private and hate to be prodded or cajoled into divulging their feelings.

Worse: Heat; sun; seaside; sympathy; mental effort; violent emotions; mornings.
Better: Fresh open air; dry weather; moderate exercise in cold air; cold bathing; rest.

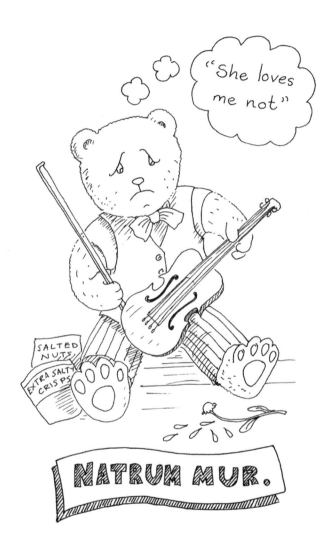

Nux Vomica

Here is another touchy customer, irritated by every little thing, such as becoming chilled, noise, light, touch or even smells can trigger a temper tantrum. They think they know best, and can be very bossy! They over-indulge, which is where a lot of their complaints begin. Whether old or teenage, they like drinking, caffeine, drugs, rock and roll. This remedy meets the typical hangover state. With zealous types, this state can come from overwork, but also from the use of prescribed drugs. They have sick stomachs, yet although they retch they cannot bring anything up. They find it difficult to pass a stool. They want lots of warm drinks and to be kept in a warm and quiet room.

Worse: Morning; Cold open air; uncovering; exertion; anger; noise; overeating.
Better: Heat; Evening; rest; damp weather.

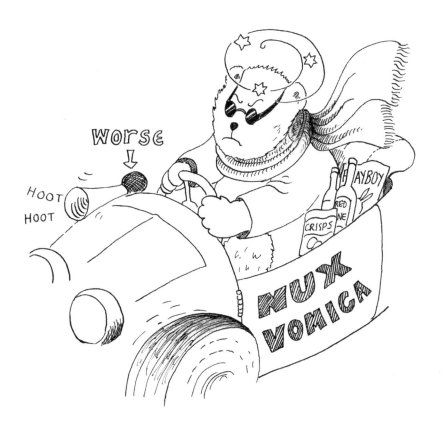

Opium

Opium and its derivatives are the best pain-killers. They are a medical doctor's trusted companion on the battlefield, in emergency situations and surgery management. Opium produces insensibility of the nervous system, drowsy stupor, painlessness and general sluggishness. These characteristics constitute the main indications for the remedy when used homeopathically. Opium may be of service when there is lack of reaction to remedies even though they are well indicated. (In this respect compare Carbo Veg.)

Complaints are characterised by drowsiness and lack of reaction, they are painless, and are accompanied by heavy, stupid sleep and snoring. Reappearance and aggravation of symptoms from becoming heated; seeks cold and is better for it. The face may have a vacant, mottled, bluish appearance. We observe contracted pupils; suppressed voluntary movements; possibly convulsions; depressed intellectual powers. There is a lessening of self control and powers of concentration and judgment. 'Thinks he is not at home; wants to go home.' The imagination may be heightened with horrid or beautiful visions, and there may be delusions that he can perform the greatest deeds. All secretions except those of the skin are checked; the skin may be hot and sweaty.

These states often originate from a great fright (such as the death of a child) or life-threatening situation such as an accident or after major surgery. The person becomes numb, insensitive and indifferent in order to survive. The situation is experienced as too much to bear, and so the person becomes insensible to what is going on, lost in their own world. They may be gentle and mild and without anxiety and fear. Nothing seems to affect them. They may laugh involuntarily.

Some conditions that may call for Opium:
Bowel obstruction (after surgery). Cerebral accident. Concussion. Constipation. Fecal impaction. Insomnia. Meningitis. Narcolepsy. Seizures. Sepsis. Sleep apnoea.

Worse: Emotions; fear; fright; shame; joy; odours; alcohol; sleep; suppressed discharges; receding eruptions; becoming warm; sunstroke; during perspiration. Better: Cold.;uncovering; constant walking; vomiting; coffee (all symptoms except trembling); open air.

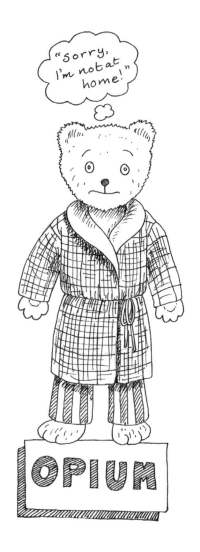

Phosphorus
This person will not show how unwell they are, and you will often see children needing this remedy playing happily with a high temperature or a stomach ache. They are easily reassured and love company; they are warm and pleasant to be with, having a sympathetic and affectionate nature. They are imaginative. As twilight draws near they may become more anxious and weak. They fear the dark, ghosts, storms or that something horrible may happen. They ask for icy drinks, or ice cream that is vomited as soon as it warms in the stomach. Often their voice is hoarse, this and most symptoms get worse in the evening. Their chest can be tight and they can have difficulty talking especially when they are out in the cold. They suffer from upset tummies, and have gushing diarrhoea that burns, and they feel sick.

Worse: Evening; lying on the left side; excitement; thunderstorms; change of weather; physical or mental exertion.
Better: Massage; company; sleep; even a short nap; cold food or drink.

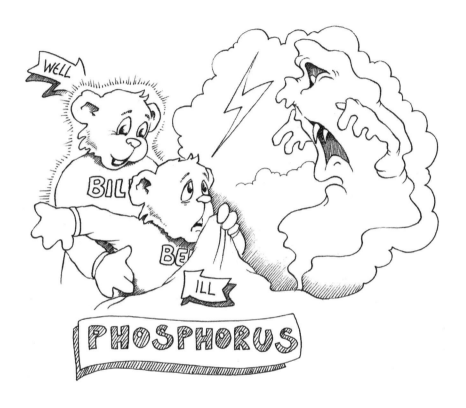

Phytolacca

A good remedy in new mothers for breastfeeding problems such as cracked nipples, blocked milk ducts, mastitis and over-production of milk. Pains are intense and radiate out from around the nipple, sometimes all over the body. The breasts may feel lumpy, stony hard, swollen or tender.

Recurrent or acute tonsillitis; dark red throat (with white spots on tonsils), worse right side; worse warm drinks, better cold drinks; pain extending to ear on swallowing.

May also be useful for headache and backache with a bruised, sore feeling, where there is a constant desire to move but all motion aggravates the pain. The person feels very cold although there may be a feverish, hot feeling in the head. There may also be shivering and a feeling of exhaustion, with restless sleep.

The person feels gloomy or fearful of death, alternatively there may be indifference to life.

WORSE: Rising from bed, motion, swallowing swallowing hot drinks, cold, change of weather, rainy weather, breastfeeding.
BETTER: Pressure, lying on abdomen or left side, cold drinks, supporting the breasts (in breastfeeding ailments), bathing, resting, warmth, dry weather.

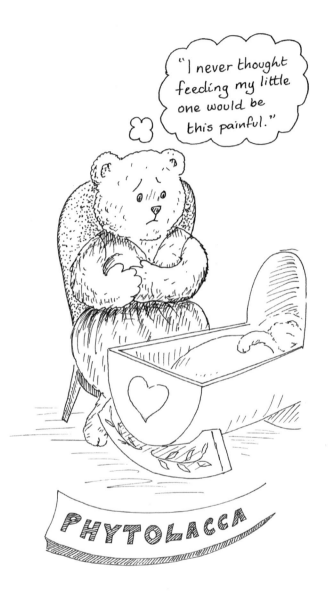

Pulsatilla

These people often feel alone, forsaken and need a friend to share with. They are affectionate, emotional, yielding and tearful; almost always better for a cuddle and kind words. They can be manipulative to get attention. A prominent feature of this remedy is the changeable nature of the illness and the person. They find it difficult to pin down their emotions and symptoms. Children can get into this condition after parties when they may have had quarrels with friends and feel left out, or have overeaten cakes and pastries. They always want lots of sympathy and cuddles and to be in their parent's bed, to be reassured when they feel alone and scared over the monsters that may be lurking in the dark. They are dependent and seem to invite a warm caress or a hug and words of sympathy. Their moods change easily. As a counterpoise to changeability, they can sometimes take one given thing to the point of fanaticism. For instance they can develop strong fixed ideas regarding religion or politics or food. Often they are upset even long after eating rich, fatty food like pork or cream. They feel the cold, yet are absolutely intolerant of any form of heat; they crave fresh air and rush to open windows. Their catarrh is thick, and yellow or green, they are prone to middle ear infections after colds, and if they get their feet wet they can gets bouts of vomiting and diarrhoea. They are usually thirstless despite having a dry mouth.

Worse: Twilight; morning; after eating; warm rooms.
Better: Cold/fresh air; cold food/drink; after a good cry; gentle motion.

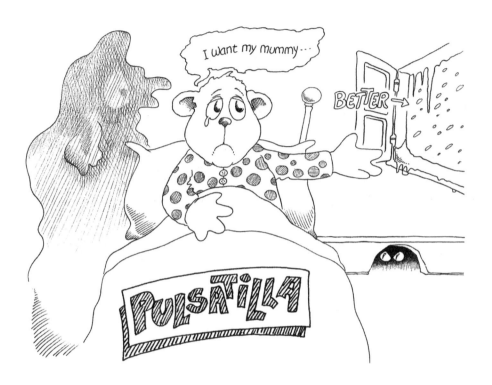

Rhus Tox.
This is a very common chicken pox and shingles remedy where the blisters look like small jellies on red plates and itch like mad, better for heat and hot bathing. It should also be the first port of call after sprains and strains and rheumatic pains that come on after being out in the cold and damp. The person aches and feels stiff, and is worse at the beginning of a movement but eases up with continued motion. Since the pains tend to return if they stop moving, they become restless. Desire to stretch, especially during sciatica, backache or rheumatic pains. They commonly have a great thirst for cold water or cold milk, and may have a taste of blood in their mouth. In stomach conditions, check the tip of the tongue for a red triangular tip for confirmation. Those needing this remedy feel unspecified apprehension at night or feel threatened, without knowing why. When in health, these people are usually family and community minded, looking after the interests of others as if they were their own.

Worse: When first moving; cold and damp.
Better: Continued motion.

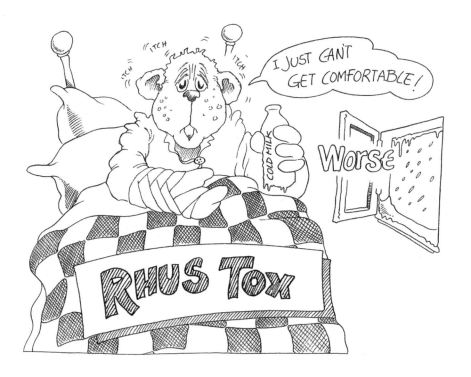

Ruta

A useful remedy for injuries to tendons, cartilage and bone surfaces (periosteum), especially in the wrists and ankles. Worth considering for sprains, fractures and especially dislocations. The injured bone feels damaged. There is an all-over sensation of lameness, especially in the limbs and joints. There may be an aversion to movement although motion brings some relief. There may also be thirst for ice-cold water.

Ruta is indicated after a difficult, prolonged labour where the rectum protrudes from the anus, particularly on attempting to pass a stool.

Disturbances of accommodation with eyestrain, followed by headache; eyes may burn like balls of fire. This may have been caused by too much detailed work.

The person feels weak and weepy, generally dissatisfied with himself and others and is inclined to quarrel. Imagines he is being deceived.

WORSE: Overexertion, injury, eye strain, lying down/lying on affected part, sitting, dusk, cold, damp, resting.
BETTER: Warmth, moving about indoors, lying on back.

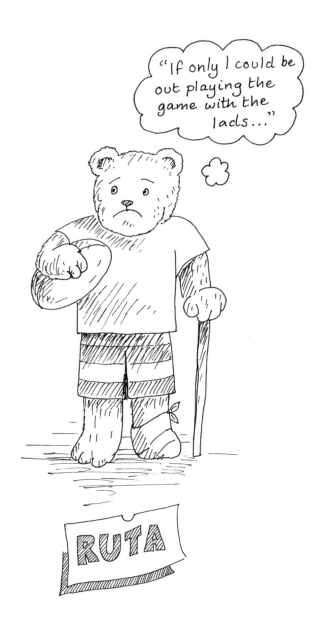

Secale

Predominantly a women's remedy and useful during labours with long or weak contractions. If the contractions stop, trembling starts. Also used to antidote the ill-effects of Syntometrine (routinely injected to speed up expulsion of the placenta) or to expel a retained placenta.

The person is extremely restless. They are very hot, though the skin feels cold when touched. They are worse for warm air; warm clothes; a warm bed; a warm room; a hot stove. They experience burning heat, like sparks of fire, and must uncover.

The person may be very thirsty for cold drinks or ice, or for milk.

The person may feel emotionally stupefied/confused. They may be restless, over-excited, raging, suspicious, shameless, mocking. Mania with inclination to bite; with inclination to throw themselves into water and drown themselves.

WORSE: Warmth and warm drinks, covering of affected parts, before and during menses, pregnancy, loss of fluids, after eating, drawing up of limbs.
BETTER: Cold bathing and cold air, uncovering, rocking, forcible extension, stretching limbs, rubbing, after vomiting.

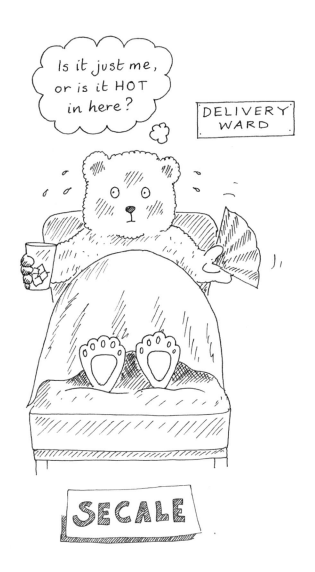

Sepia

These people, usually women, suffer from stagnation of their energy on all levels: they have 'turned off'. This has come about because of overwork, over-care of children and family duties. At the emotional level their tender feelings have turned off, mentally they are absent-minded, thinking is difficult, while at the physical level their systems are slowing down and they suffer congestions; circulatory disturbances (hot flushes during menopause); constipation; bearing-down sensations (especially in the womb); emptiness in the stomach; total lack of energy, dullness. Aversion to sex: no desire, no orgasm. They tend to be chilly and are worse for becoming cold. If she can find the get-up-and-go she is better for violent exertion, running and dancing.

Finding that they have become unable to give or receive love and affection, they want to be left alone. This state may trouble them, especially when it relates to their lack of love of their children, or it may have settled into a chronic state in which they have become incommunicative and defensive. They weep when speaking of their state, being overwhelmed by sadness, but without the ability to think or communicate clearly. Like Natrum Muriaticum they may be worse for any attempts at consolation, warding off affection with aggression. Fault-finding, fretful, sarcastic, spiteful, striking, and much worse before menses.

Worse: Cold weather; wet weather; before; during and after menses; sexual excesses; pregnancy; miscarriage; menopause; standing; mental exertion; before thunderstorm; after first sleep; afternoon; during and right after eating; drinking milk. Aversion to fat.
Better: When busy; dancing; open air; warmth; sitting with legs crossed; for eating. Craving for acids; vinegar and chocolate.

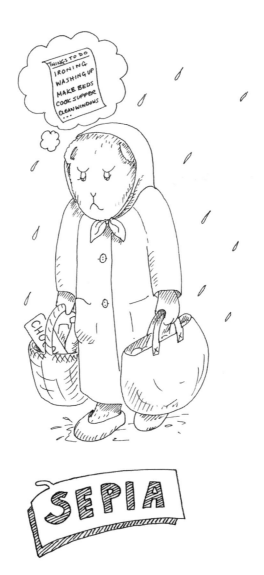

Silica

Children and adults needing Silica are prone to lingering infections for instance in the site of wounds, scars, rotten teeth and vaccinations. They also find it difficult to throw out splinters; they yield to foreign bodies, until they are give potentised Silica to wake up their dormant resistive powers. In Silica persons, these intrinsic 'resistive powers', although quiescent, are great: enough, for instance, to stimulate the body to throw out embedded shrapnel from old war wounds. We see this in the mental sphere also where the physical properties are mirrored. Silica people are outwardly mild and seemingly yielding, yet have an inner resistance; they stand firm, and may obstinately maintain their point of view. They do this because of inner determination as much as a concern about what others may think about them: that the image they project should be perfect. Adults and also children can give us a refined, almost aristocratic impression: inwardly assured (hard) yet outwardly polite (yielding). This characteristic can remind us of Staphisagria. Whenever there is a possibility of their image being lost, for instance while appearing on stage or meeting new people, or at the time of exams, Silica people develop tremendous anxiety with a great fear of failure. Silica may appear like Lycopodium, because Lycopodium also has lack of confidence. But in Lycopodium, it is whether they are capable of doing the action that bothers them, while in Silica it is their image that must be protected at all costs. Silica people are always conscious of the impression they are creating. This can make them fidgety, or they may give rehearsed answers, giving the impression that they are formal. They are apt to be overly conscientious about trifling matters: great at calculation, work with precision, obsessive attention to just one detail. Silica comes in after prolonged mental overload; people who push themselves to the utmost with stubborn perseverance to fulfil a specific task.

In children there may be delayed development and growth; slowness of recovery; late in developing relationships. Loss of hair in intellectual children, especially when under stress at school; premature balding.

Worse: Becoming cold; cold drafts; damp; uncovering (especially the head); bathing; checked sweat (especially on feet). Sensitive to nervous excitement; light; noise; jarring spine; change of moon; night; mental exertion; during menses; after vaccination; milk; alcohol.
Better: Warmth; wrapping up well; after profuse urination.

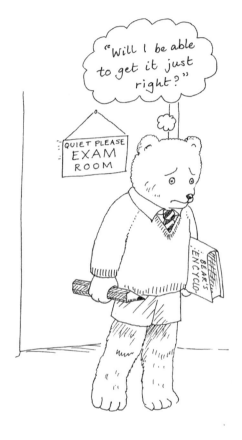

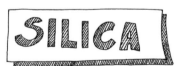

Staphisagria

Those needing Staphisagria are morbidly sensitive to being cut, injured, and to feeling insulted. These people avoid quarrels at all costs because such unseemly acts are below their dignity. If you let the Staphisagria person speak you may be amazed at their sense of righteousness, which can reach such a height that they feel morally superior to others, yet they feel that they must deign to accept a lower authority in order that the wheels of socially acceptable 'good form' run true. As written, they are exquisitely sensitive to being injured and this includes their sensitivity to the rudeness of others that cuts them to the quick. They fear losing self-control as they perceive this gross behaviour as being below their dignity. They are mild mannered, they will not fight, and may accept authority to an extreme degree. For these reasons these people are prone to suffer from ailments from suppressed emotions and anger.

Staphisagria people are often of a romantic disposition, and therefore they are easily disappointed. They may have nostalgia for the beginning of a love affair when things were sweet, yet they stay in the relationship because of the fear of rocking the boat and awakening anger. As well as being romantically minded, they tend to be sexually oriented. Intruding sexual thoughts may drive them to masturbation. They are apt to have strong sexual fantasies and can only fall sleep after masturbation. Sometimes there will be a history of sexual abuse.

Extreme sensitiveness to touch: genitals, warts, haemorrhoids, eruptions, injuries. This is a major remedy after operations where catheters and anaesthetist's tubes have 'invaded'. Trembling from suppressed anger or nervous excitement. Constant swallowing from suppressed emotions. Pains that move into teeth. Blackened and crumbling teeth. Cystitis after coition and after catheterisation. Pain in bladder or abdominal colic after surgical operations.

Worse: Emotions; grief; vexation; indignation; quarrels; insults; mortification; suppressed feelings; sexual excesses; touch; cold drinks; lacerations; morning; afternoon nap; night; tobacco (which they may crave).
Better: Warmth; rest; breakfast.

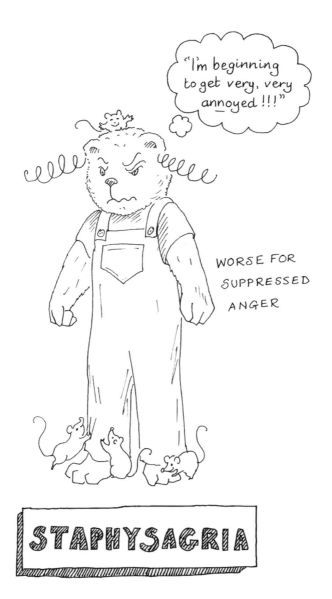

Sulphur

The most noticeable thing about the character that may need this constitutional remedy is they have a strong tendency to be scruffy. Even if they have just had a bath, they still manage to look unclean. There are two types of Sulphur: one is outgoing, strong, solid and the other quiet, skinny and unsure of themselves, but both types take little care of their appearance. Both types can have red, dry, flaking skin, which can itch and burn and is worse from washing. They often have dry, unruly hair. They are hungry and thirsty, particularly in the late morning and will crave strong flavoured food, fat and sweets. Milk disagrees with them. They commonly have diarrhoea which has them jumping out of bed for relief first thing in the morning. They may be constipated. Their runny nose makes their skin sore. They feel the heat and often stick their feet out of the bedclothes at night.

They are very untidy and they hate to throw old things away because they think that all their possessions are better than anyone else's. They like to tell everybody how to act in their life. They want to know all the answers, are really inquisitive, and can be very demanding, yet they do learn quickly. They are impatient, hurried and restless, wanting to do things themselves. Teenagers can be lazy and full of their own opinions. They will lap up any praise you may give them. They love debating for the sake of the argument and winning so as not to feel put down or shamed. A peculiarity: they hate to stand.

In summary, Sulphur falls into two types: the introverted philosophical, theorising individual who wants to penetrate into the deep secrets of the universe, and the outgoing practical, yet nonetheless idealistic types who have many ideas but no time, or it's too much trouble to realise them. Both types can be self centred and egotistical, appearing to have a very good opinion about themselves, yet just below the surface they are very sensitive to criticism, scorn and insult. Both types are warm-blooded and will want doors and windows open. They have burning pains and sensations of burning and itching with redness of the skin, especially around their orifices. They are apt to have offensive discharges that burn the skin over which they flow. Desire for sweets and spicy food.

Worse: Heat; 11 a.m; at night; damp; sunshine; scratching.
Better: Movement; open air; dry warm weather.

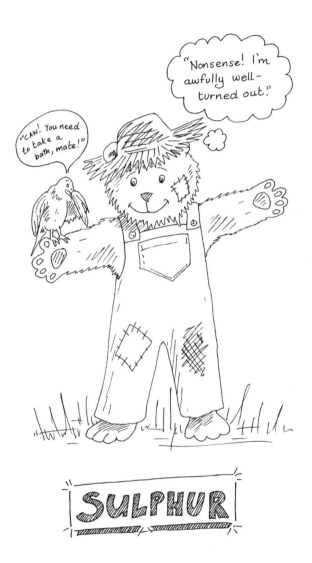

Symphytum

A useful remedy for speeding up the healing of fractures. But first see to it that the bones have been correctly set! Non-union of fractures (compare Calc phos). Also useful for mechanical/blunt trauma injuries such as blows, bruises and eyeball injuries (such as an infant thrusting its fist into its mother's eye) and cartilage injuries, and for old but still painful injuries to cartilage or periosteum. The fracture site feels very sensitive (may be felt as a pricking pain) and there may be residual bone pain long after the injury has healed . Also irritable stumps after amputations, when there is soreness of and pricking pains in the bone. Phantom pains.

The person may feel alternately cold and feverish all day. When cold they will want to wear more clothing. The person feels generally weak and miserable, and may dwell excessively on past disagreeable occurrences.

WORSE: Injuries, blows from blunt instruments, touch, motion, pressure.
BETTER: Gentle motion, warmth.

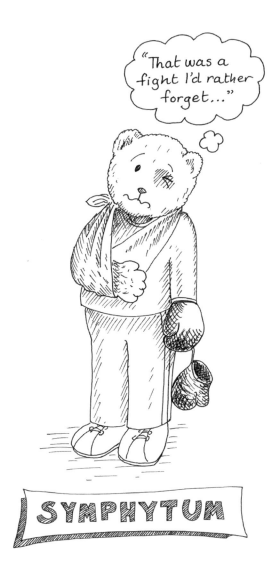

Further information

Suggested Reading
Some good books to get you started:
The Complete Homeopathy Handbook · Miranda Castro
Homeopathy - Medicine of the New Millenium · George Vithoulkas
Pointers to the Common Remedies · Margaret Tyler

For more advanced readers wanting a grounding in homeopathic philosophy:
The Genius of Homeopathy · Stuart Close
The Principles of Art & Cure · Herbert Roberts
Spirit of Homeopathy · Rajan Sankaran

For those wanting to consult a brief text book of homeopathic medicines:
Materia Medica · Dr SR Phatak

These books and more are available from Alternative Training:
Alternative Training · www.alternative-training.com
T: 0800 0439 349 or 01453 765 956 · E: info@alternative-training.com

Finding a homeopath
For information about finding a professional homeopath in your area contact:
www.findahomeopath.org.uk

The Society of Homeopaths · www.homeopathy-soh.org.uk
11 Brookfield, Duncan Close, Moulton Park, Northampton NN3 6WL
T: 0845 450 6611 · F: 0845 450 6622 · info@homeopathy-soh.org

Alliance of Registered Homeopaths · www.a-r-h.org
Millbrook , Millbrook Hill, Nutley, East Sussex, TN22 3PJ
T: 01825 714506 · F: 01825 714506 · info@a-r-h.org

Faculty of Homeopathy · www.facultyofhomeopathy.org
Hahnemann House, 29 Park Street West, Luton, LU1 3BE
T: 01582 408680 · F: 01582 723032 · E: info@facultyofhomeopathy.org

Homeopathic Medical Association · www.the-hma.org
7 Darnley Road, Gravesend, Kent, DA11 0RU
T: 01474 560336 · F: 01474 327431 · info@ the-hma.org

Homeopathy Helpline

If you need urgent homeopathic advice you can contact the homeopathic help.
This is a premium rate number for professional advice, the call duration is usually
10 minutes. The charge is around £1.50 per minute:
Homeopathic Helpline · www.homeopathyhelpline.com
T: 0906 534 3404 · E: fran@homeopathyhelpline.com

Homeopathic Pharmacies

While a number of the remedies mentioned in this booklet are obtainable from Health
Food Shops and some Chemist Shops, the potency supplied is usually 30c. In order
to obtain a comprehensive selection of remedies it is best to contact a Homeopathic
pharmacy that provides a 24 hour mail service. The pharmacies listed below will
respond swiftly to a telephone order.

Helios · www.helios.co.uk
97 Camden Road, Tunbridge Wells, Kent TN1 1QR
T: 01892 537 254 · E: order@helios.co.uk

Ainsworths · www.ainsworths.com
38 New Cavendish Street, London W1M 7LH
T: 020 7935 5330 · E: enquiries@ainsworths.com

Nelson · www.nelsonshomeopathy.co.uk
73 Duke Street, Grosvenor Square, London W1M 6BY
T: 020 7629 3118 · E: pharmacy@nelsonbach.com

Homeopathy Courses

Want to know more? Why not take a course in homeopathy? There are plenty to choose from. The School of Homeopathy offers part time attendance courses as well as professional home study courses from beginner to practitioner level. Taster, Foundation, Introduction into Practice and Practitioner Diploma courses are available. The Practitioner Diploma course leads to accredited professional practice. The home study courses are run along Open University lines. No prior medical knowledge is required for any of the courses, as we provide this in-house. The School is well known for its high standards and creative approach. For a prospectus please contact the School of Homeopathy.

School of Homeopathy · www.homeopathyschool.com
Orchard Leigh, Rodborough Hill, Stroud, GL5 3SS
T: 0800 0439 349 or 01453 765 956 · E: info@homeopathyschool.com

For a contact list of other homeopathy courses contact the Homeopathic Course Providers Forum: www.hcpf.org.uk

Get Well Soon